# IRISHMEN DON'T CRY

*A Medical and Emotional
Journey with ALS*

# RICHARD P. FLYNN

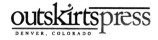

DENVER, COLORADO

Irishmen Don't Cry
A Medical and Emotional Journey with ALS
All Rights Reserved.
Copyright © 2013 Richard P. Flynn
v4.0

Cover Artwork, "A Passion For Skiing," by Maggie Connors.
Photography by Peter Harris Studio.

Outskirts Press, Inc.
http://www.outskirtspress.com

ISBN: 978-1-4787-0950-3

Outskirts Press and the "OP" logo are trademarks belonging to Outskirts Press, Inc.

PRINTED IN THE UNITED STATES OF AMERICA

# Acknowledgements

This story began in sorrow, moved on to hope, and is ending in joy. To thank everyone would be impossible. I would have to include everyone in my life. I will do my best.

Harvard Vanguard, The Veterans Association, Massachusetts General Hospital's ALS clinic and Compassionate Care of Falmouth have all given me immense support.

The three amigos, Barry Hickman, Jack Manley, and Billy Allen, have been with me every week for years now. I could never repay them for this tremendous loyalty. Thanks to Al Butters, my classmate from grade school, who has rekindled our relationship. He even brought Sister Mary Black, our fourth grade teacher, to lunch. She helped turn us into men. Bob Sawtelle, Joe Plunkett and Jimmy Roddy have been very helpful and steady in their support. I want to thank Butch Donohue for pinch running for my mother. Thank you Carol Walsh and Judy O'Hara for being good friends. Matt and Denise, the owners of Fishbones, and Chrissy, the owner of Siros, have been amazing in their support. Thank you Maggie for doing my cover and being a lifetime friend. Thanks to Michelle for her love and support for what seems like forever. Peter G has always been there for me. That won't be forgotten. John McQueeney, another lifelong friend, has even made a few trips from Texas. Thank You. Earl, even though you are bed ridden, you always take the time to inquire about me. Thank You.

Carolyn, my administrative assistant, has labored through every word of this book with me. And believe me it was literally word by word towards the end. She has true talent, and you will be reading a book by her someday. You have defined compassion for me, Thank you.

My wife, Nancy, swept into my life in 2002. She was the kindest, most caring, intelligent and beautiful person I had ever met. Little did we know then that she would become my guardian angel. Four short years later I was diagnosed with this dreadful disease. She never blinked, immediately taking on the challenge. She has been there every step of the way, creating the nurturing environment that allowed me to persevere and write this book. It could not have been done without her. I love you and thank you!

Richard Flynn

# Table of Contents

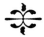

# Foreword

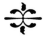

*Irishmen Don't Cry* is a heartfelt and enlightening journal of one man's journey with ALS, Lou Gehrig's disease. This is more than a typical autobiography. It teaches so many lessons. The lessons may be ones we all should know but hearing them in this book only adds something to each of our lives. To be able to hear how in one simple day life can be changed forever. In this very eloquently written story, Richard brings us back to the initial diagnosis seven years ago. A trip to the doctor for his finger, thinking it was simple nerve damage, resulted in a diagnosis of a very serious neurological disease. He includes his therapists and doctors notes and letters in his journal. His interpretation of these visits with his use of humor keeps the topic light in spite of the seriousness of the disease.

In spite of a predicted two year life expectancy in 2006, Richard has beaten the odds. He writes this book as a love letter to his wife, Nancy, but it's a love letter to all of us in a way. We will all take something different away from Richard's journey, which includes stories from childhood to present day experiences living with ALS. It reveals to us that no matter how different we are, we are all vulnerable. It inspires you as you read how he accepts his challenges with courage. It really does prove that whatever each of us may face we can overcome if we have the right attitude. Seven years later Richard is still proving this by living his life each day to the fullest. He speaks of his losses of mobility and speech in the book, but recognizes that his mind is still sharp. He chooses to wake up everyday and be positive, even grateful and not feel sorry for himself. In fact he feels he has been given a gift in a way, a time to reflect on his journey.

Its a story that will stay with you long after you finish reading it. Richard's powerful journey will be etched in your heart forever. It will teach you many things that you will be able to apply to your own life. It will have you laughing and crying at different times. You won't want to put it down. Just remember, attitude and spirit are everything. This Irishman chose not to cry but to take this courageous journey instead.

Richard presently lives in Marina Bay with his wife, Nancy. He is working on his second book. Richard plans to finish the book by Christmas 2013.

Carolyn Arrigal

# The Beginning
## 11-3-06

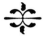

*Diagnosis: Muscle weakness*

*Nurse practitioner Leslie Hunt refers this right-handed man for evaluation of left-hand pain with weakness over the last few months. He has noted difficulty tying his shoes and buttoning his pants and has some cramping of the left hand. Months ago, he noted some stumbling with the left leg. There has been no stepwise deterioration in function.*

The sun was bright and strong as I valeted the car and walked into the hospital, apprehensive, yes; worried, no. A few more MRIs and scans, and I should be fine. Probably slept on the nerve or something. Worse thoughts never crossed my mind. Was I prepared for what was to come? No. I walked through the office door upright and confident.

*Impression: This patient has months of painless weakness of the left arm with normal sensation and slightly brisker reflexes on the left than the right. Motor neuron disease is the most likely diagnosis. Will look for motor neuropathy and immune-mediated neuropathy with appropriate blood tests and EMG. I will also get another neurological opinion with a neuromuscular expert to make sure there is no treatable disease we are overlooking, and then he will follow up with me.*

After getting a thorough examination, I said, "What do you think, Doctor?"

His answer tore through me. "Mr. Flynn, I think you may have a serious neurological disease. We don't know for sure. We will do more tests."

"What's the best prognosis?" I asked.

"Two to five years," he answered.

So much for feeling upright and confident. The ride home seemed infinite. Thoughts raced through my head like meteors. What do I do? How do I deal with this? What do I tell Nancy? I stared blankly ahead. Tears welled up in my eyes as I struggled with my own mortality, and then all of a sudden I found strength and said to myself, "Irishmen don't cry."

That night Nancy and I went out to dinner with our neighbors. I got drunk and told them Nancy and I were to get married in Italy, and I would put them all up. Of course it never happened. I did get married in Europe later on, but that's a story for another day.

The next morning, after I woke up half hung over, my mind started galloping again. What would I do? Would I retire? How does one prepare to die? So many things to think about. It then struck me: I won't change a thing. I will lead an active life no matter what. At that point I made a commitment to myself: *I will bring people together and show them how to die with grace and dignity.*

## One Week Later: Second Opinion

*Diagnosis: Neuropathy*

*The patient is referred for a second opinion by Dr. Pilgrim for evaluation of possible motor neuron disease. The patient is seen with his significant other, Nancy. They verbally report and bring in documents that indicate*

*Nancy has power of attorney and is a healthcare proxy, and we have total freedom to speak about medical matters with Nancy. I sent the documents for scanning. The patient's history is that beginning this past summer, without a specific precipitant noted, the patient gradually noticed weakness of his left hand, which has progressed. He also has noticed some stumbling with his left leg when he exercises on a treadmill. He thinks his right-hand writing is a bit sloppier, and he admits over the past couple of years on occasion he has an individual difficulty swallowing. A couple of years ago he had neck pain radiating to the right upper arm. He was left with some mild neck pain. In recent months and years, he has had low back pain that occasionally radiated down the back of the leg at least to the knee, which is unremarkable. He denies any arm pain.*

*On exam, the patient appears healthy and comfortable. His pupils, his eyelids, and his eye movements are normal. The face moves symmetrically. The speech is well articulated. He swallows saliva without difficulty. Palate and tongue are midline. There is mild atrophy of the interosseous muscles and FDI of the left hand. No other atrophy is apparent. All other muscle groups in the left hand, left arm, right arm, and legs are all symmetrical and intact. The patient was taken for EMG nerve conduction predominantly to evaluate the left arm. The EMG did show abnormalities quite consistent with findings such as a small number of fasciculations in other muscles and some polyphagia in other muscles that are soft minor nonspecific findings that require some caution in interpretation. There also was a significant chronic denervation in the left L5 pattern consistent with the history of sciatica. A clear electrical diagnosis of motor neuron disease was not forthcoming.*

*The impression is that most likely the left-leg symptoms are the result of old sciatica. We indicate that the left arm symptoms may be an atypical ulna neuropathy. What would be atypical would be the absence of parathesias and also atypical would be these additional soft EMG findings in other muscles; however, at this time there may be good news that the hardest and most definite abnormalities in the arm are all simply consistent with an ulna neuropathy, rather than motor neuron disease. The patient and his significant other do seem to understand that there is a degree of uncertainty in the diagnosis and they do accept that the passage of time will likely clarify the matter. The patient does not report a prominent history of leaning on his elbow, but he will make sure he does not lean on this elbow, and he will determine whether he will follow up either with me or Dr. Pilgrim in approximately one month. A copy of this report was sent to Dr. Pilgrim and his primary care clinician.*

Now uncertainty. What a roller coaster! This could be the ALS, or it could be an elbow nerve. Nothing to do now but wait. I hate to say it, but its worse not knowing. Meanwhile, the progression continues in my hand, arm, and leg. The hand is starting to feel more like a club, but believe me, slow is better than fast. What a way to have to treat a disease! Wait until it turns out to be something else or gets worse. Either way, it's like water torture, but I'll wait and hope for the best. After all, Irishmen don't cry.

## Five Months Later: March 30, 2007

*Diagnosis: Muscle Weakness*

*The patient reports continued progressive weakness in the left hand. In addition, he says that he has to use the hand as a claw when he is pulling things sometimes. There has been no neck pain. He says that when riding in the car, he will sometimes lean the elbow on the windowsill, and it feels like there is something emanating from the left elbow.*

*Impression: This patient's weakness is progressing. I told him to place the left arm inside the pillowcase with a pillow in place to try to protect the ulnar nerve further, in case this disorder is related to a left ulnar nerve. I will see him again in three months. The differential remains motor neuron disease versus ulnar neuropathy.*

The diagnosis seems to be slowly moving toward ALS but then again, who knows? I may luck out. I struggle to define what is going on in my life. The definition of *progressive* in the dictionary reads, "Becoming more severe: describes a disease that becomes more widespread or severe over time. Synonyms: Powerlessness, defenselessness, helplessness, impotence."

Powerlessness? Holy cow, as Harry Carry would say, particularly for a guy who has always been in control. The answer turned out to be simple. I would take control of the situation and find the courage to cope through my passion, skiing.

A passion can be anything. It can be the girl next door; in fact most often it is the girl next door. It could be sports. It can't be booze; that wouldn't work, although it could be the history of beer or wine.

My passion just happened to be skiing. Let me tell you how that happened. The year was 1962, and I was a junior at Roslindale High School. Roslindale High School was not Weston High School, although my mother thought it was. We did not have Saturday ski trips or vacation ski trips, but we did have Bob Sawtelle, part comedian, part class clown, and part friend, and it was his idea to plan a ski trip. Little did I know it was just him and me and two chicks. On a snowy Friday, we left on the bus for North Conway, Bob and I, the two chicks, and a bottle of vodka.

In late afternoon, we arrived at the inn. Soon we were joined by a busload of guys and gals from Boston. It was a wild night for a seventeen-year-old. I hope my mother isn't turning over in her grave as I write this.

The next day we set off skiing with only enough money for one set of equipment and two lift tickets. After the wild night, the girls refused to ski. I'm not sure they were even talking to us, so Bob and I took turns coming down the mountain, even though his foot was a ten and a half and mine was a nine and a half. That, folks, was the beginning of a mad love affair with skiing.

Skiing has kept me from being a couch potato and possibly a drunk. Now my passion will have to carry me through this journey. I will need to feed my passion as this health issue progresses. You know, sometimes Irishmen are too dumb to cry.

## Two Months Later: June 25, 2007

*Diagnosis: Muscle weakness*

*The patient comes for follow-up for muscle weakness in the left arm present for about one year. He finds it impossible to button things with the left hand, but he has really noted no extension of his weakness beyond the left hand.*

*Impression: This patient has progressive weakness of the intrinsic of the left hand without other weakness. The reflexes are brisker on the left. The syndrome best fits motor neuron disease, but the pace of deterioration in the absence of spread of deterioration to the other extremities argues against the usual picture. I will continue to follow him. I have extended the interval form three months to six months. He knows to come sooner if there is deterioration.*

Now one year has passed since I first noticed a weakness. The craziest thing is I can't tell people what I might have, because I look so healthy. I'm still walking fine. I feel perfectly healthy. Some days

I feel as if this is not really happening or it is some sort of perverted joke. Guess what? Time to plan a ski trip. Feed my passion and, I hope, starve the disease. Italy again! Tenth straight year! Nancy and I will go in January to Cortina D'ampezzo, the jewel of the Dolomites. I will see my Italian friends, and we will gorge ourselves on wonderful food, a combination of Italian and German. Regional cooking at its best. What better way to cure a cold or whatever?

Why would an Irishmen cry when he could eat?

## Six Months Later: December 5, 2007

*Diagnosis: Neuropathy*

*The patient returns in neurological follow-up. He has had weakness in the left hand that began in mid-2006. There has been no pain, no weakness anywhere else, and no swallowing difficulty.*

*An EMG performed in 11/2006 showed chronic denervation in the left L5 myotome, consistent with sciatica, mild, mostly symmetrical, small sensory potentials in the hands, raising the question of a mild underlying generalized neuropathy, and the strongest abnormalities in the left arm were compatible with left ulnar entrapment at the elbow.*

*The patient saw Dr. Wilkins in second opinion, who thought that the patient's hand syndrome was due to an atypical left ulnar neuropathy.*

*Impression: This man has weakness of the left hand with increased reflexes on the left side compared to the right. The pattern best fits motor neuron disease. His course has been present for about a year and a half without weakness in the right arm, the legs, or the neck, making this a very unusual variant. I elected to repeat his EMG.*

Wasting away is right, but slowly, nevertheless. Thank God Italy is just around the corner, less than three weeks away. I dream of skiing Faloria, Cristalo, Lagazua, and Alta Badia. Rifuguos, mountain retreats that offer food and lodging, around every corner, it seems, and the best meat ragu in the world. God bless the Italians! No matter what happens, they persevere through it and survive. There's a lesson to be learned there.

More tests. I guess that's just how it's going to be. I'll take them all, and then I'm off to the mountains of Italy. *Ciao!* Italians probably cry a lot!

## January 22, 2008

*Diagnosis: Neuropathy*

*The patient returns for neurological follow-up for weakness in the left hand since mid-2006. There has been no pain. He has no other weakness.*

*The patient has a disorder, mainly the median, but also the radial nerve, of unclear etiology. I would like to get an EMG. One is scheduled for next week, and then we will get another opinion.*

*The long history without weakness outside the left arm argues against motor neuron disease.*

A year and a half, and they are just as confused as I am. Not an exact science, that's for sure. They don't know much about the disease. They don't even know if it's one disease or a number of diseases that came together. My luck! What a great health history the Flynns have: heart disease, cancer, brain aneurisms, bad veins, alcoholism, and now possibly ALS, if the doctors can ever make up their minds.

Late January. Italy was great. Skied all one day with an Italian instructor who had climbed K-2. Skied from mountain to mountain for days on end. Went to Corvara and Sud Tyrol, one of the most beautiful places on earth. I came back all in one piece. My reflexes and balance are still intact.

*Phone call: "Mr. Flynn, we have taken this as far as we can. We need to refer you to someplace with more resources. Do you have any preferences?"*

Thank God I'd done my homework. I chose the ALS clinic at Mass General, soon to be named the number-one hospital in the country. I also chose Dr. William David, a graduate of Albert Einstein School of medicine. How's that for instilling confidence?

Surprisingly I got what I asked for, and the referral was made. This Irishman is really confused now, but he still won't cry.

## Date February 12, 2008

*Re: Flynn, Richard*
*MR#: 2581306*

*Dear Dr. Pilgrim:*

*Thank you for referring Richard Flynn for a consultation regarding hand weakness.*

*Assessment:*

*Richard Flynn is a sixty-two-year-old male with two years of slowly progressive upper and lower motor neuron findings primarily limited to the left upper extremity, but also involving the right hand to a lesser degree. His abnormalities conform to a segmental distribution. These observations are most compatible with a diagnosis of amyotrophic lateral sclerosis*

*(ALS). Without the benefit of primary involvement in his nerve conduction/EMG studies, we draw this conclusion with slight reservation. We discussed this with Mr. Flynn and his girlfriend today. I met with the patient for the first time as part of his consult today with Dr. David. The patient comes in today to have received confirmation of his diagnosis of ALS. He and Nancy have expected the outcome. We discussed the natural progression of ALS, and based on his history and current symptoms, he may be in the grouping of slow to moderate progressors. We discussed the issues that we know improve survival and can help maintain strength.*

Well, you wanted clarity, big boy; now you have it! They don't ever really tell you that you have ALS. They just sort of slide into in. My mother warned me: be careful what you wish for. Now I pretty much know, but I've already set out my goals and plans on how to live my life. The test now is to see how I do. The progress has been so slow. The journey hasn't really begun yet. There will be a lot of detailing of symptoms in the future, but somehow it is a bit easier for Nancy and me to know what we are dealing with for certain. Nancy has been tough and will need to be even tougher from now on. She is my angel. Maybe Irishwomen don't cry either.

# The Middle

Now the journey has begun in earnest. I laugh. I feel like Lewis and Clark, but now I can address the fact that I have a fatal and debilitating disease. No one ever said it would be easy. I have led a charmed life in many ways. Championship at age twelve, a good education, a great childhood, business success, and money. I even managed to get a decent handicap in golf, and most of all, I became a great skier.

Now I will be dealing with doctors and hospitals for a long time. God help them, they don't know what they're in for. I am determined to make this disease sorry it attacked me. I know that sounds foolish, but that is how I feel. Irishmen aren't afraid of a good fight!

The nightmares had been there for years, but now they have increased in severity. They are no longer enemy ambushes. Those I knew were from PTSD. These nightmares are different. In one I killed someone, and the police were chasing me. I would wake up in a cold sweat, feeling totally out of control.

In order to cope with the nightmares, I started meditating. After about a month, the nightmares went away. After about three months, I stopped meditating, and guess what? Some of the more recent nightmares came back. I guess deep down I preferred a good action flick. No one ever said this Irishmen was smart!

Now that the worst is basically confirmed, people are beginning to ask questions. For some reason people have a morbid interest in death, as long as it doesn't involve them. The questions begin: how are you going to prepare for death? Are you afraid of dying? Well, it's simple. I've been preparing to die my whole life. Am I afraid of death? No. I am more afraid of not living the rest of my life to its fullest with the gifts God gave me. Am I afraid of how I die? Not really, but I do know that suffocating is not pleasant. They will probably have me full of morphine anyway.

I made plans to wrap up my business by April 1, 2008, and I did. I also began to make plans to retire, which I did officially in November 2008. Fifty-five years of working. Not working would require an adjustment that could be harder than dying. I could still walk and talk and had the entire use of my right hand, so I know it will be only a matter of time before I take a part-time job just to keep busy.

I do feel different now. I have fewer ups and downs. Life is not the same as it was before. I try not to get angry over petty things, and I value and respect other people more than ever. Life can be crazy enough without something like this happening, but I will cope with it. My life has been forever changed, but that can be turned into a positive. I have good friends, and even my dog supports me. The process slowly continues. It won't paralyze my spirit, which will live on long after I am gone. Life is precious, and I realize that fact more now than ever.

The progression of paralysis marches on. Sometimes it feels as though my insides are turning to butter. There is a tendency to feel like I am trapped inside my own body. I now realize that I am. That issue will be dealt with, even if I have to piece Humpty Dumpty together again.

All the king's men tried to help Humpty. Maybe they can help me stay together. There is no established way to deal with this disease. Half the time I am winging it. That's o.k., though, because at times, it opens more doors to explore. This experience is really an expedition and a journey. A journey doesn't have to be painful. My mind can create all sorts of wonderful things. I am going to put it through the test. I am determined to have a positive outlook and be a positive influence on others. It's that time again; even Irishmen need help at times!

## Early Spring 2008

It's been almost two years now. The progression is what it is. It will not speed up or slow down. It will remain at the pace it started. The doctors are sure of that. I will deal with it like a continuum. I won't consider it a fatal disease. I will treat it like I am simply moving from one phase to another. At some point it will get ugly. Right now that seems a long way away. I will treat it like any other disease. It progresses, and I'll deal with it. I have a feeling the next few years will tell me a lot. The key is to keep my spirits up and not get grumpy. Time will tell if I can do it.

During my life's time I have been totally independent, even stubborn, some would say. I will deal with this issue independently, no matter what is happening around me. It doesn't feel like time is running short; therefore I will start working on my bucket list. No Italy this year. In the early summer, I will set up a trip to Sun Valley, land of Sonja Henie and John Payne. "Sun Valley serenade, here I come."

Ketchum, Idaho: Hemingway lived there, and there are plenty of good restaurants. Notice how I got back to food again. They say that Idaho potatoes are great. I will find out. I wonder if there are many Irishmen in Idaho.

## May 20, 2008: Physical Therapy

*Mr. Flynn returns to Neuromuscular/ALS clinic today for follow-up care. Nancy accompanies him on his visit. He reports slowly progressive left-hand weakness, which is interfering with some functional activities, such as buttoning shirts and pants, cutting food, etc. He is also an avid skier and would be interested in having some sort of splint fabricated for next ski season, to enable him to hold a pole in his left hand.*

*Mr. Flynn reports no notable weakness or problems with his legs and can ambulate, climb stairs, and ski without difficulty. He reports that he gets regular exercise, and I encouraged him to continue doing so.*

*We discussed a number of things, including adaptive devices, to help with functional activities. I gave him information regarding large-handled silverware, buttonholers, and adaptations for pants zippers, including websites where such equipment may be found. He will go online and obtain the things he thinks will be helpful.*

*Amy Swartz, PT*

The spring passed slowly into summer. I am not depressed, I don't think. I am still upright and active. Progression is still slow, but it seems as though I am always waiting for the other shoe to drop. I'm not depressed, but I do get sad at times. I feel sad about leaving the people I know and the places I've seen. It is not a fear of death, but sadness about leaving so much behind. When one is active and healthy, you take all these things for granted. I, of course, thought I was invincible, and maybe I will be in the long run. People talk about what horrible childhoods they had. Even without any father, who died when I was nine, I had a wonderful childhood. We were safe and played daily in the woods of West Roxbury. We even played softball at night on an abandoned farm. My mother could really hit, even in her house coat, and Butch Donahue would pinch run for her. She had bad legs. Butch went on to become the state champion. He got his start with my mother. As we got older, we would play ball at Billings Field every day and all weekend.

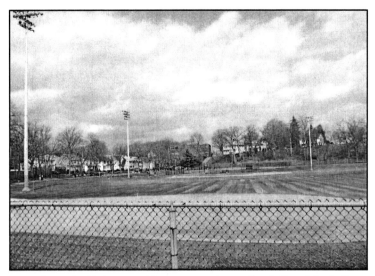

*Billings Field: hours and hours spent playing baseball and football.*

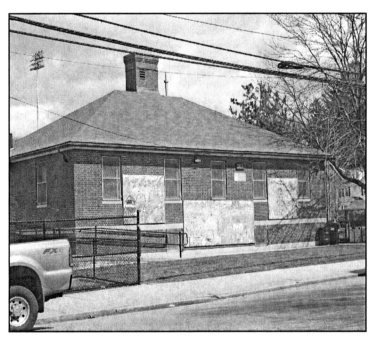

*Richard and Jay McCarthy used to sit there changing and talking about playing football for the NFL.*

It's midsummer now, time to book Sun Valley. This trip I've been thinking of since the 1950s.

## August 2008

Palmer penmanship has all but ruined my handwriting. It was never very good, but now it is worse and at times illegible. I decided to retire. I knew it was time. A few days later, I went to the Social Security office. After a long wait, they let me in. I explained that I wanted to retire, which I thought would be simple. After a few more minutes, the woman said, "If you retire today, I will have to turn you down," so I reached into my bag of 1960's activism and said, "Let me speak to your supervisor. I've been working since I was nine years old, and I am not going to be turned down."

The supervisor came over, and I said, "What do I have to do to retire?"

She said, "You have to be out of work for two months before you can apply."

"O.K," I said. "I'll retire now, and give me a date to come back two months from now," which they did. Before I left I looked at the woman and said, "That was simple, wasn't it?"

Two months later, my retirement came through. Five months later, the disability came through, not a nightmare, but not very efficient either.

Retirement. This was not the original plan. My dream was to retire and spend six months in northern Italy and six months here. I pictured myself at seventy years old walking through the streets of Cortina in a snowstorm with skis bouncing on my shoulder. I will still travel, but I have to be within reach of my doctors. So much for being an Irish legend in Cortina!

## December 23, 2008: Physical Therapy

*Mr. Flynn returns to Neuromuscular/ALS clinic with Nancy. He reports no significant change in left hand and forearm weakness and atrophy. He remains independent in all mobility; some activities, such as buttoning shirts and cutting food, are more difficult due to left hand weakness.*

*Patient continues to exercise at the gym five days/week. He also downhill skis every weekend.*

*He had received short-term OT to have a splint fabricated to enable him to hold a pole in his left hand. He reports that this is working well.*

*We discussed the importance of maintaining shoulder ROM, hamstring and heel cord stretching. He appears to be on a very adequate exercise program. Mr. Flynn will meet this morning with our clinical nurse practitioner and physical therapist regarding functional recommendations. In many respects he appears to be doing quite well. He will be skiing up in New Hampshire later this week and will be traveling to Idaho in early January 2009 for another ski trip.*

January came fast. Before I knew it, I was sitting in a ten-seat airplane going over the mountains and landing in Sun Valley. Going to new places is great. I feel like I am a child experiencing everything for the first time. Sun Valley did not disappoint. So much was recognizable from the movie.

The skiing was challenging, and I knew it would be. I also found a new hero, a ninety-two-year-old man, all hunched over, who skied every day.

I knew I would eventually get back to food. Their restaurants were great. Fresh trout caught that day, and at the Pioneer, the best and biggest Idaho potato I've ever had. The rock massage at the Sun

Valley Lodge was impressive.

Our room overlooked the skating rink where Sonia Henie performed. After a great week, Nancy and I vowed to be back. We barely scratched the surface of this gem.

## April 14, 2009: Physical Therapy

*Mr. Flynn returns to Neuromuscular /ALS clinic today for follow-up care. His primary issue is still left hand and arm weakness, which he feels is progressing. He reports he is having difficulty with functional tasks, such as cutting meat and working with buttons and zippers, but has a buttonholer zipper pull that works well for him and is considering a rocker knife when needed. We discussed a few other assistive devices, and he will obtain the necessary items as they are needed.*

*Mr. Flynn reports that he is going to the gym regularly and skied all winter, though the season has ended now. He has no difficulty with exercises at the gym, though he has backed off on some of the weights due to his left arm weakness.*

*Overall, Mr. Flynn seems to be managing very well.*

## April 14, 2009

I am still upright and going strong. I never thought that I would be able to be this strong against this disease. This is almost three years now since the onset. The strangest thing is I don't feel bad. So far this has been cataloging only minor progress as the symptoms slowly advance. It's hard to imagine what it will be like when it turns ugly at the end. For now I am just living my life the best I know how. No cures seem to be on the horizon; therefore, I'll do the best with whatever I have left.

## August 18, 2009: Physical Therapy

*Mr. Flynn ambulates without an assistive device and is independent with all mobility. His primary complaint to this point has been left hand weakness.*

*Today he notes that his weakness has progressed and he is unable to flex his fingers or form a fist, even passively. With passive range of motion testing, he has significant contractures of his finger and wrist extensors, with passive movement just beyond neutral and pain at end range. We discussed the reason for the contractures, as well as a plan for stretching to maximize his range of motion with heat and prolonged stretch. If stretching does not improve his ROM significantly, I would highly recommend a course of intensive OT and possibly splinting. His contractures are significant and are causing him considerable discomfort.*

*Mr. Flynn also has right posterior ankle/calf pain that he thinks may be his Achilles tendon. It has been very painful and has altered his gait, but he feels it is getting better slowly with icing. His posterior calf is painful to palpation over the Achilles (in the approximate area of the musculotendinous junction) but not painful at insertion. Mild stretching of the Achilles does not cause any pain. His neurologist has recommended ibuprofen, and I agree with this plan, along with icing and gentle stretching. We discussed different stretches, including towel stretch and stair stretch, stressing the importance of prolonged, non-painful stretching. If the pain does not significantly decrease in the next week or two, I strongly recommend a course of outpatient PT for treatment. He will continue icing, add stretching, and will call me if it doesn't improve in the next two weeks.*

It's not enough that I have this insidious disease, but now I have a strained Achilles tendon. I'm falling apart! I'm sure it's just from driving too much. Am I the biggest loser or what? Progression is still slow, but the hands are deteriorating even more. I suppose it's only a matter of time before I lose my mobility, but I will keep fighting it. We are having Thanksgiving in New Hampshire by ourselves. A nice turkey, small but delicious. I am doing the cooking still. Notice how I got back to the food again. Time for a gut check and get ready for Christmas. We will be skiing at Cranmore with Nancy's grandchildren. The last time I was at Cranmore was 1962. *Buon Natale*, Irishmen!

## November 2009

*Dear Dr. Miller:*

*I recently had the pleasure of seeing Mr. Richard Flynn, a patient of yours, in following the MGH ALS Center. We last saw Mr. Flynn on August 18, 2009.*

*Since that time he has noted a slight deterioration in his right hand. He has been experiencing right arm cramps and has observed fasciculations proximally in the right arm. His handwriting has deteriorated. He has not noted any symptoms in his legs. Getting up and down stairs has become slightly more difficult, though he is not aware of any specific weakness. He did go skiing last week. He has a sense of easy fatigability; nevertheless, skiing was not compromised. He has experienced occasional cramps in the left leg.*

*He continues to be free of other symptoms. He has not noticed any difficulty with speech or swallowing. He has had no weight loss. He denies shortness of breath. He has had no excessive daytime sleepiness or orthopnea.*

*At the time of his last visit, we discussed the possibility of starting Celexa. Mr. Flynn did acknowledge some signs of irritability; however, he decided not to start taking the medication.*

*He had some specific questions regarding the upcoming stem cell trials in Atlanta. We reviewed this as well as some other ongoing research endeavors. Mr. Flynn also inquired about physical therapy exercises for his left hand. He also has some concerns about his handwriting as well as his future ability to drive.*

No really bad news heading into Christmas, just a steady progression. As you can see from the results below; some things are getting more difficult.

Speech: 4 = Normal speech processes
Salivation: 4 = Normal
Swallowing: 4 = Normal eating habits
Handwriting: 3 =Slow or sloppy; all words are legible
Cutting Food and Handling Utensils (patients without gastrostomy)
2 = Can cut most foods, although clumsy and slow, some help needed
Dressing and Hygiene: 2 = Intermittent assistance or substitute methods
Turning in Bed and Adjusting Bed Clothes: 4 = Normal
Climbing Stairs: 3 = Slow

Other than my hand, I still have my balance and mobility. I will ski my way through Christmas and into January. Some people think I'm crazy, but this is the only way I know. Sun Valley is looking forward to seeing this crazy Irishman again. I can't disappoint her; she is far too beautiful.

## Buon Anno 2010

As I head into the New Year, they are talking about my being depressed. Some people have called me crazy, but never depressed. If I am depressed, I'm the happiest depressed person I know. I decided not to take the antidepressants at this time, so here I go to Sun Valley. I am basically skiing with one pole now, because the left hand can't support one. That's fine; it's all in the feet and legs anyway.

I skied a lot and spent more time in Ketchum, a great western town. Had a few drinks in the Ducin Lounge at the lodge. Their charcuterie was magnificent. It is getting more difficult to ski challenging conditions. I know that next year I'll have to go to an easier mountain. Deer Valley came to mind. I'll have to work on that.

We took a sleigh ride at night, and I actually didn't freeze to death. Boy, those horses smell!

Dinner at a remote cabin was delightful. It became harder to think of not coming back, but I'll move on and work my way through my bucket list.

This Irishman has got to get to Ireland too; otherwise I won't feel complete. Something seems to be drawing me there. It seems almost spiritual in nature. I still have an interest in western Ireland and the Aran Islands. Tough living. I wonder if the Irishmen over there cry.

## May 2010

*Dear Dr. Miller:*

*Over the past few months, Mr. Flynn has developed some progressive symptoms. His right hand continues to weaken, and he is having difficulty writing. He has also been experiencing occasional cramping in his right hand.*

*He has noted episodic leg soreness, which is new. He has been experiencing some cramping is his thighs and his calves approximately three to four times a week. Stretching will alleviate the cramps. Although he is unaware of any specific weakness in his legs, he has noticed fatigue when going upstairs. This is not respiratory in origin. He feels that his legs will fatigue as he ascends, and he is now using his arms to assist him in climbing. He has no difficulty walking on flat surfaces. He was able to ski this past winter, though he was limited in this regard. He was unable to ski two consecutive days. Additionally, he would limit each outing to two to three hours. Previously, he was able to ski for much greater lengths of time.*

*Mr. Flynn was taking citalopram for two to three months. He reported improvement in his mood and a decrease in irritability; however, he feels that this medication gave him nightmares. As such, he stopped the medication approximately three to four weeks ago; subsequently, his mood declined and he became more irritable. In retrospect, Mr. Flynn has suffered from post-traumatic stress disorder. He has had nightmares for several years, although he believes that the citalopram accentuated these nightmares. This is somewhat uncertain. His sleep has been disturbed. Previously, he was also taking Zolpidem. He is not taking this medication at present. After some discussion, we suggested that he restart the citalopram as well as the Zolpidem.*

As you can see from the chart below, things are starting to deteriorate more:

Speech: 3 = Detectable speech disturbances
Handwriting: 3 = Slow or sloppy: all words are legible
Cutting Food and Handling utensils (patients without gastrostomy)
1 = food must be cut by someone, but can still feed slowly.
Dressing and Hygiene: 2 = intermittent assistance or substitute meals

Turning in Bed and Adjusting Clothes: 3 = somewhat slow and clumsy, but no help needed
Climbing Stairs: 2 = mild unsteadiness or fatigue

I can feel my dependency slowly increasing. That is a natural progression with this disease, but it still feels very strange. I am not used to relying on others for anything. This is an unnatural transition.

They have put me on a mild medication because they think I am getting a bit grumpy. No shit, Dick Tracy!

I am looking forward to summer now. We'll go to the beach house in April this year. Life goes on! So far I've been able to handle the bumps in the road, but now it appears to be getting rocky too. The good news is at least I am not in denial. I am dealing with this head on. Only God knows how it will turn out.

## July 2010

*Dear Dr. Miller:,*

*I recently had the pleasure of seeing Mr. Richard Flynn, a patient of yours, at the MGH ALS Clinic.*

*Since that visit, Mr. Flynn has noted advancing weakness of his left hand. He has also observed evolving right-hand weakness. He has had increasing difficulty with fine finger movements in the right hand. He has difficulty squeezing bottles. He continues to experience episodic hand cramping on the right side.*

*He has not noticed any significant symptoms in his legs. He gets occasional leg cramps in his left leg. He feels that his legs fatigue easily. He does experience some difficulty going up stairs; however, he is unaware of any specific weakness in his legs. He has noted some cramping in his jaw.*

*Mr. Flynn and Nancy both suspect a mild degree of speech dysfunction. Mr. Flynn states that he is speaking a bit slower and stiffer. He may also be experiencing some mild dysphagia. He has had a few choking episodes. This has not been a major issue. For the most part, he eats foods of all consistencies and he has not lost any weight.*

*He denies any significant respiratory difficulties. He occasionally gets winded; however, he denies orthopnea or excessive daytime sleepiness. He does take an occasional nap.*

*He has been sleeping better. He has been taking citalopram with benefit. He has a prescription for Zolpidem, but takes this only rarely.*

Summer is moving quickly. The hands are worse, and I'm starting to feel it in the legs. I'm going forward with Deer Valley. We will be staying at the Stein Eriksen Lodge, which is on the side of the mountain at 8,200 feet. Skiing should be tremendous! I look forward to January. The pictures on the Internet don't do it justice, I'm sure. I'm lucky to have very good friends, and they are giving me plenty of support, but I realize that this is a battle I must fight myself. I realize that when push comes to shove, we are all alone in this crazy mystical dance called life. That will never change. I realize how fortunate I have been. I won't spoil it now because of some silly disease. I salute all those who have forged their way forward for me. My commitment to persevere and survive is nothing compared to some who have come before me. My respect and thanks to all of you.

Speech: 3 = Detectable speech disturbances
Swallowing: 2 = Dietary consistency changes
Handwriting: 2 = Not all words are legible
Cutting Food and Handling Utensils (patients without gastrosto-my): 2 = Can cut most foods, although clumsy and slow; some help needed
Dressing and Hygiene: 2 = intermittent assistance or substitute methods
Walking: 3 = Early ambulation difficulties
Climbing Stairs: 2 = Mild unsteadiness or fatigue
Dyspnea: 2=Occurs with one or more of the following: eating, bathing, dressing

Christmas is approaching. I am experiencing changes in speech, swallowing, and handwriting. They have changed my diet to a softer consistency. This is for a man who loves fine dining. No way! This is put on hold until after the holidays and January.

Deer Valley exceeded expectations. As soon as I arrived, I had an amazing wild boar chili. It did not disappoint. One thing about Utah to remember is they do not know how to make a martini, even at the Stein Eriksen Lodge.

From 8,200 feet, you could ski down the mountain or take a lift up; we did both. Unfortunately at this time my upright skiing started to take a turn for the worse. I could still ski fine, but I had trouble getting off the lift and fell a few times. Still felt great, but I could sense that I was getting close to the end of my upright skiing. Nevertheless I skied into the spring without a major mishap. I guess I have always had angels looking over me, and the best part is that they are Irish angels who ski well!

## March 2011

*Since his last visit, he has noted more weakness in his legs. He has been having more trouble getting up the stairs. In fact, he fell down the stairs about a week ago. He hit his head and briefly lost consciousness. He was disoriented for about an hour, but since then has noted only mild tenderness of his head. Otherwise, he has not had significant headaches or confusion. He also notes worsening weakness in his arms since last visit. He occasionally has choking with liquids and solids. He has noted subtle changes in his speech. He wakes up often at night, but citalopram is helping. He denies morning headaches, excessive somnolence. He experiences cramps in his legs three to four times week and occasionally in his right hand. Mood has improved with citalopram.*

*Assessment/Plan:*

*Mr. Flynn is a sixty-five-year-old right-handed gentleman with ALS. His course has been slowly progressive, and he now has developed some left leg weakness since last visit. Safety with gait and stairs is now a concern. His FVCs had been stable in the 90s since February 2008 but last FVC was lower at 69. Subjectively, he is doing well from a respiratory standpoint: we will repeat FVC today*

*We will have him see our multidisciplinary team today, including our physical therapist, to address difficulty with stairs and possibility of AFD and chair lift for stairs. We will also have him see one of our nurse practitioners today and check FVC. Form for disability placard was filled out today.*

Of course I knew it would happen eventually; I have started falling. The worst was on the stairs, and I lost consciousness for a minute. This is disturbing but not insurmountable. I also fell in my kitchen and lay in my own urine for two and a half hours. Thank God Ron from CCALS came and rescued me. It is time to read the book of Job again, which will make me feel more fortunate. Poor old Job; every time he turned around, the crap was hitting his fan. My misfortune has been slower developing. The shoe is getting looser. It hasn't fallen yet. I skied forty days this winter, but I fear that was the last of my upright skiing. I'm using a cane now and have to have assistance going upstairs and walking. This was expected. I am not letting it get me down. I have been fitted for a leg brace that will help prevent tripping and falling. It's time to enjoy the summer and get a good tan. My spirits are up and always will be. There's some work to do around the beach house, and I will make sure it gets done.

July Fourth will be bonfire time; we are planning on a large, neat, Irish bonfire. My daughter is getting married in August, and we are excited about it. My goal will be to dance with my daughter. Other than that, it will be a normal summer at the beach with Nancy and Lexi. I am still working out and will continue to do so until they drop me in the hole. I am getting tired now, so I will talk to you during the next installment. God Bless!

## June 21, 2011

*Visit Note:*

*Mr. Flynn has noted a continuous progression in his symptoms. His legs have continued to weaken. He has significant difficulty with stairs. He has installed a chair lift in his house. He has suffered two falls since March. On one occasion, his dog pulled him too fast while walking. On another occasion he tripped going up a stair. His arms have also continued to weaken, particularly on the right. His left arm has minimal function.*

*Mr. Flynn has also noted a significant change in his speech. He is still quite understandable, though he has suffered progressive difficulty with articulation. He still experiences difficulty with swallowing, although intermittently. He occasionally will choke on thin liquids. He has no difficulty with solids.*

*His mood has been good on citalopram. He continues to be free of any respiratory difficulties. He will be receiving overnight breathing assistance starting this Friday.*

*We spoke with Mr. Flynn and Nancy about a variety of issues. We met for approximately forty-five minutes, the majority of which was spent in counseling and coordination of care. We will check CBC and liver functions today as the patient continues on Rilutek. We will recheck pulmonary function tests. We would like for Mr. Flynn to be seen by our clinic physical therapist, speech and language pathologist, and nurse practitioner. Fall prevention will be key.*

One thing of note did happen this summer. I had a tapas dinner with Billy, Sharon, and Nancy. We decided to take that long-awaited trip to Ireland. Nancy set up all the details. Two weeks later, we decided to get married while we were there. I love impulse buying. We arranged the ceremony to be at the Cliffs of Moher. The ceremony was to be performed by a monk from the Aran Islands. It will be an ancient Druid ceremony, featuring earth, air, fire, and water. We are eagerly looking forward to that. I am walking with a cane, but I will need a wheelchair for longer walks.

Time feels so valuable to me now. I will continue to bang away at my bucket list. Who knows? I might surprise myself. In any event, I hope all those bloody Irishmen in Dublin and County Clare are ready for us. Billy is learning Gaelic as fast as he can. Wait till he finds out not many people speak Gaelic in Ireland. I don't think he cares. He'll talk their ear off anyway. I am ready to immerse myself in Irish culture and will write again after I get back.

## September 27, 2011

Speech:2 = Intelligible with repeating
Salivation: 3 = Slight but definite excess of saliva in mouth; may have nighttime drooling
Swallowing: 3 = Early eating problems—occasional choking
Handwriting: 0 = Unable to grip pen
Cutting food and handling utensils (patients without gastrostomy): 1 = Food must be cut by someone, but can still feed slowly
Dressing and Hygiene: 2 = Intermittent assistance or substitute methods
Turning in Bed and Adjusting Bed Clothes: 2 = Can turn alone or adjust sheets, but with great difficulty
Walking: 2 = Walks with assistance
Climbing Stairs: 1 = needs assistance

## October 2011

I have returned from Ireland in one piece. God knows how that happened! The trip was wonderful. We toured southern and western Ireland with our own driver, just the four of us. Dublin was great, a real vibrant city. Galway was even better, because of its small size and intimacy. Very Bohemian for Ireland.

We got married on the Cliffs of Moher. Billy almost killed himself pushing me up the cliffs in the transfer chair in the pouring rain. We never did see the Cliffs of Moher. Maybe next time. Brother Dara performed the ceremony. Afterwards we all had a pint at McGann's in Doulin. After that we changed and had a wonderful after-wedding meal, followed by traditional Irish music. Brother Dara came, as did our driver, John.

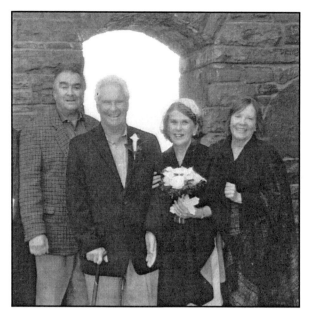

*Wedding party at O'Brien Tower, Cliffs of Moher.*

The landscape was beyond belief, as were the people. As an added bonus, the food was great, because of a ten-year boom in the economy. The result was many new restaurants and chefs.

We saw Ireland and got married to boot! We are already talking about going back.

It's November now, and I will not be skiing upright. I have made arrangements to ski disabled, but so far there is no snow. It looks like disabled skiing will start in mid-December. I'll be there; you can bet on that. By the way I was able to dance that dance with my daughter. If it were to happen today, I would not be able to.

December came quickly. I skied disabled and took to it right away. It is exactly like skiing upright; all the techniques are the same. This is fantastic; I can continue to ski in spite of my condition. There will be no major ski trips this year. I will concentrate on skiing at Loon. I can't believe how exhilarating it is. We are already talking about maybe racing next season.

## January 3, 2012

*Mr. Flynn returns today for follow up. He was last seen on September 27, 2011. Since that time, he has noticed slow deterioration in speech, lower extremity weakness, and dysphagia to liquid and solid. It is harder for him to rise from a seated position. He fell about three weeks ago in the bathroom. He tripped, catching the right foot. He did not sustain any injuries. He was not able to get up from the floor, but he alerted his wife through a mobile alert, and she was able to help him. The right hand has become significantly worse. Turning over in bed has become difficult. Breathing has been stable. He lies flat at night. He denies morning headaches. He does not fall asleep spontaneously throughout the day. He stated that he is eating well. His weight has remained stable after losing some weight in September. He has some drooling at night but not much during the day. He is unable to cut his food but can still bring food to his mouth with utensils. His FVC was 61% of predicted on June 11. He is a bit irritable and wonders if his citalopram can be increased.*

*He lives in Quincy with his wife. His house has two floors. Chair lifts have been installed to get him up and down the stairs. There are grab bars in the shower. He uses a cane and transfer chair. He does not use his walker much, because his left hand is too weak to grasp it. He wears a left AFO. He just received a motorized scooter that he intends to use in the spring/summer.*

*Louis Tramontozzi, M.D.*
*Neuromuscular Fellow*

As you can see from the medical notes, my condition is deteriorating. I still enjoy a normal lifestyle, though. The breathing is what I worry about the most. It is 56%, now from a high of 103%. Pretty soon they will have me use a breathing machine at night. I will do whatever keeps me going. Life is too precious to give up on it. There is no give up in an Irishman. We are all too stubborn.

## April 30, 2012

*Patient Name: Flynn, Richard P.*
*MRN 2581306*

*Date of visit: April 3, 2012*

*Mr. Flynn returns today in follow-up. He was last seen on January 3, 2012. He continues to note progressive weakness, worst in the right hand and legs. He's primarily using a power chair for mobility. His speech is becoming increasingly dysarthric. He uses an iPad with communication application quite well. He has bilateral AFOS but does not use them much, now that he is walking less.*

*Appetite feels good, though he feels he has lost a little weight. He has some choking, worse with thin liquids. Increasing problems clearing secretions. Weight is down five pounds since June 2011.*

*The Zoloft is being tolerated well. His mood is good, and he hasn't suffered any side effects as he did on other antidepressants. Mr. Flynn maintains a very active life. He has recently been traveling in the Caribbean and plans a trip to Ireland with his wife this summer. Over the winter he kept busy with adaptive downhill skiing.*

*Recommendations:*

1. *He will meet with PT regarding possible right hand splint to maintain range of motion.*
2. *Referral to social work for assistance in hiring personal care attendants*
3. *Letter for the airline stating he needs to bring the BiPap with him for his trip to Ireland in July*
4. *Speech for ongoing weight loss and language impairment*
5. *We began a discussion about a feeding tube and discussed that if he is inclined, we will recommend making this transition before swallow and breathing impairments become severe. We discussed the potential risk and benefits.*
6. *Check CBC and liver function tests as he continues on Rilutek*
7. *Pulmonary function tests will be rechecked.*

ALS is like a high handicap in golf. All of a sudden it will rear its ugly head. Here is where I stand now. I'm just back from a trip to St. Thomas and St. John. The trip was great! The food was not. They need to work on that. I now have two leg braces, a hand splint, an elbow splint, and a breathing machine at night. I have resisted it up until now, but they have lined me up for a feeding tube in July. The ALS is entering its uglier phase now, but I have angels on my side. Barry and Billy have been coming every week. Billy Allen takes me to a movie most of the time. Billy was one of the best athletes ever to come out of Massachusetts. He was a three-sport all-scholastic in high school and started three sports at Boston University, captaining the football team. After college he played three minor league seasons for the Red Sox. He hates it when I compare him to the golden Greek, Harry Agannis.

Barry Hickman, West Roxbury's own golden boy, and I have lunch and a couple bottles of wine at Fishbones every Thursday.

Barry later played football at Wake Forest, and minor league professional football, but not before returning one of the most exciting last-second game-winning punt returns in Boston schoolboy history.

Recently we have been bringing Jack Manley along, another friend. Jack was an excellent all-around athlete, but he always preferred teaching and coaching. I have started to call it Wednesday at the movies and Thursday at Fishbones. The guys won't go anywhere else, because they like the pretty waitresses. The commitment they have made to me is beyond belief.

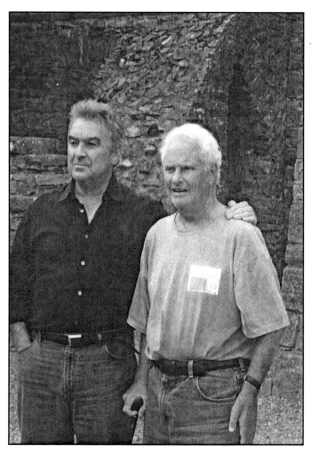

*Wednesday at the movies critics, Billy Allen and Richard.*

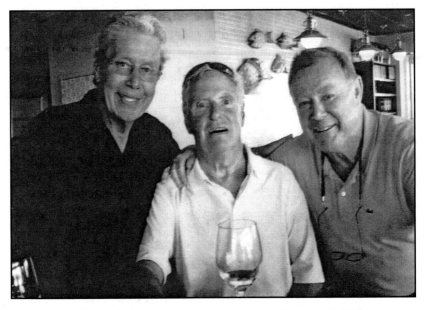

*Jack, Barry and Richard, the spirit-ual club at Captain Fishbones.*

My chief angel is Nancy; somehow she has managed to deal with all of this.

I now have several personal care assistants, one who shaves and washes me in the morning. I also have PT, which is great. There are various other speech and swallow nurses as well.

This month, April, another angel showed up on my doorstep. This is Carolyn; she is with me most afternoons, five to six days a week. She is my administrative assistant and does most everything I need to get done. She even makes hermit cookies for us! I don't know how she works out the pressures of attending to her own family and me, but she does. She is even helping me with this book.

This month she and I started going to Humarock at the end of each week. We had lunch at the Bridgeway Restaurant. We have now started a Friday afternoon tradition at the Bridgeway. It's amazing. At times it's like the crossroads of the south shore. I see old friends and people from grammar school. Of course the food is good, and the bartenders are perfect. It's a great way to start a weekend.

P.S. There is no shortage of Irishmen at the Bridgeway.

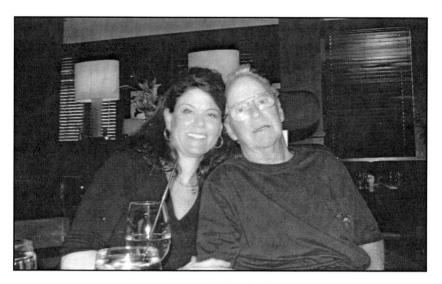

*Carolyn and Richard at lunch.*

## July 2012

I am now six years into this dreadful disease. They want me to have a feeding tube inserted before my breathing gets worse. I delayed this move, but I will have the procedure done tomorrow.

*A/P: Mr. Flynn is a sixty-seven-year-old male with ALS, who has been symptomatic for approximately six years. He is wheelchair confined. He continues to have worsening weakness, both limb and bulbar. He has support at home now with staff coming in as well as PT. The major plan is for a feeding tube tomorrow, although he can continue to eat a soft diet for now. He does have some worsening trouble with salivation, and we discussed possible interventions such as a suction device and pharmacotherapy*

Don't ever let anyone tell you that this operation is easy. I have a super high pain threshold, and this was a real pain in the you-know-what. They had tubes in every orifice of my body, and then they asked me how I felt. I thought, *You must be nuts*, and I said, "How the hell do you think I feel?" The best part was what they did to my stomach; they moved it into place and attached it to my abdominal wall. Eventually it will adhere to scar tissue. They proceeded to poke a hole in my belly, through the abdominal wall and into my stomach. All this was done on local anesthesia. They then installed a plastic tube, which was probably put together by minimum-wage workers in Taiwan. Thank God this was all done at Mass General Hospital.

If the doctor tells you that this procedure is merely uncomfortable, don't believe him. It is very uncomfortable at best, and painful at its worst.

All in all everything went well. Two days later, my dog, Lexi, was nosing around the operation site and seemed upset. Sure enough, she was right; I had an infection. The nurse sent me back to the hospital. They quickly took care of that.

Guess what! I'm leaving for Ireland again at the end of the month. I'm sure I'll be fine by then. If not, it doesn't matter. I'm going anyway. A simple local site infection can't keep a good Irishman down.

Billy's daughter came up with the idea for this second trip to Ireland. It was planned around the Galway races, which are a lot like our Kentucky Derby. Billy rented a house in Galway for Sharon, Lura, and Hardy. Nancy and I stayed at the Park House Hotel. Fabulous!

We went back to the Cliffs of Moher one day, since we hadn't seen it on the day we got married, because of the pouring rain and lack of visibility. We got there this year, and the skies opened up for twenty minutes, but we could see them. Another day we went to the shrine at Knock. Just to update you, I wasn't cured.

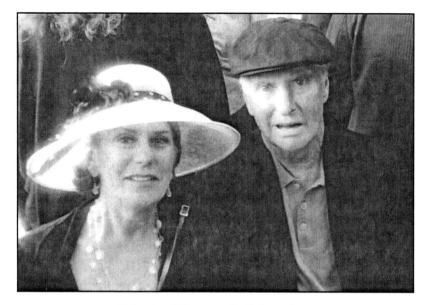

*Richard and Nancy at the Galway Races.*

We spent two days at the races. If I had known the prize for the best hat was $25,000, I'd be touring the world entering hat contests.

The final two days, we spent exploring Galway city. It was great! This is a very cosmopolitan and bohemian city. The food and people were an added treat. I had a motorized scooter, which worked out well. Guess what. I didn't see a single Irishman cry.

*Mr. Flynn comes to clinic today in a transport wheelchair, adjusted the footrests to lower height. He now requires moderate assistance with transfers out of the wheelchair. At home he uses a motorized w/c and also has a roll-in shower and lift into the house. Wife asked me to call Bernadette (OT at the VA) to get flu appointment with him for next week. He would like to get w/c van from VA. I gave them a RX for a wheeled commode chair. PT reports receiving a split bed rail from the VA.*

*Progressive weakness in arms and legs (especially left) continue. He has severe dysarthria and only a few words are understood with repeating. He has an iPad with communication application. He has moderately limited ROM of left shoulder and left elbow flexion.*

*Pat Andres, DPT*

It is October, and I'm into heavy-duty equipment now. I have a motorized wheelchair on order. A handicapped van just arrived, and that makes everything a lot easier. I also have a lift that I will eventually need to get in and out of bed. I call it T-Rex; it hovers above the bed like some menacing prehistoric beast. I'm still leading my normal, stubborn, Irish life.

## November 2012

Our second trip to St. Thomas/St. Johns came quickly. We spent five nights at St. Thomas, Frenchman's Reef, and three nights at St. John, Caneel Bay. The food was lousy again. I figured out what part of it is. They don't use salt and pepper when cooking. Everything tastes neutral. Either that, or my taste buds are gone. Caneel Bay was a joy! It has to be one of the most beautiful, peaceful, and discreet places on earth.

Friday night, in that peaceful atmosphere, I had my first sense of death within me. It was as if I could feel my insides wasting away. Nancy blames it on the two rumrunners, but that wasn't it. The next morning I looked at my arms in the mirror. They looked like the grotesque disfigured arms of a death-camp survivor. Emaciated. Not encouraging, but I will deal with it by doing more physical therapy. Resistance always helps. I think my dog, Lexi, can smell the wasting away. She is always at my side now, particularly if there is no one else with us. Just like Nancy, Carolyn, and my other friends, she is a rock. I knew that dog had some Irish in her heritage.

It is the day after Thanksgiving. Thirteen trails are open at Loon. Time to check on disabled skiing. We called, and they are going to open December 15, 2012. We have a few weeks to get ready. We now have a new dog, Paris, who should be called Paris Chanel. One of these days I expect her to come around the corner in a little black Coco Chanel dress. I will have to get her ready for the snow. That should be fun; she is a wild one. She is a hundred percent Parisian. No Irish in her!

This will be my second year in adaptive skiing. I bet I'll be the only person skiing with a feeding tube. Maybe I'll hook it up to a water camel. Irishmen do get thirsty, you know.

I plan to go up the mountains around December 7, 2012. I have a small lift I need to bring up there. I call it mini T-Rex. It's not as menacing as the larger one.

I now have great difficulty talking. Carolyn and I are on a race with time to get this book on paper. At some point in time it will become word by word through a computer.

I also lost my ability to taste food. It is strange, though, I still have a sense of each taste in my brain. It's not the same, but it makes it easier. I also still have a feel for the texture of food. It is amazing how that helps, so I still enjoy eating to a point. All is not yet lost. I think it is time now for a good Irish stew.

The paralysis is worsening. The van helps me get places I wouldn't ordinarily be able to reach. The doctors said the ALS would not increase or decrease, but this year things seem different. It is as if there has been a wild collision of symptoms. I have now lost the use of my legs, arms, hands, taste, and smell. My voice is almost gone. I gave a speech in September in which I mentioned the loss of these functions: September 27, 2012.

*Today I'm here to speak about CCALS. I will start with what it is not. Medical! Doctors have catalogued symptoms for 160 plus years with no cure. Drug companies have had the same length of time with no cure. The government, lots of red tape, and no cure.*

*What is CCALS all about? People associate CCALS with equipment for patients, and it does supply hundreds of thousands of dollars' worth of equipment for ALS patients every year.*

*What CCALS should be known for is Compassionate Care. It deals with the physiological, emotional, and spiritual side of the disease. That is the true worth of CCALS, a bright light in what could be total darkness. CCALS helps you realize that you can lead a normal life, even if you don't have the use of your arms, legs, or voice.*

*Before I took a trip one time, Ron said to me, "Wear your disease like a badge of honor," so while I was in Europe, someone asked me what was wrong with me. I said proudly, "People (over here) call it motor neuron disease. In America it's called A.L.S. I prefer Lou Gehrig's."*

*To my fellow ALS survivors out there, remember you are very special! Wear your disease like a badge of honor! If you do, we will never again be the target of a tasteless joke in an insulting movie.*

*God bless you all; God bless CCALS, and God bless Lou Gehrig! Thank you!*

In it I mentioned how one can live a normal life even with these challenges. Normal has, of course, changed. It is changed for good, but I will still plug away at it. Sometimes I feel like Sisyphus, rolling that huge rock up the peak. I think my mountain is less steep and more forgiving than his. Ironically, as my mobility decreases, it is offset by an increase in technological mobility. I thank Compassionate Care, Mass General Hospital, and the VA for this. They have helped enormously! I am in a Mexican standoff with the disease. It could have been so much worse so much sooner. Sometimes I wonder if God may be Irish.

## Early December 2012

Two weeks from now I will be skiing disabled. This should be a great year. I should be faster and smoother than ever. I have to remember to call Jack and reserve a time at the mountain. I wonder if performance-enhancing drugs would work. Wouldn't that be a riot, getting thrown out of disabled skiing for using performance-enhancing drugs? Now that I think about it, I don't need to. I have enough energy running through my veins; even my cardiologist agrees with that. Besides, the only drug a good Irishman needs is a room temperature pint of Guinness.

## Christmas Season 2012

My next doctor's appointment isn't until after the New Year. That allows me to enjoy my favorite time of the year, the holidays. Even when I was not home physically, I was always there in spirit. I remember one Christmas in Ethiopia. We got drunk on Hurricanes, paid the horse-drawn-carriage driver five dollars, and raced the carriages through the streets of Asmara. The military police loved it. That was almost as bad as the time I brought a horse into a private Italian club. I still can't believe the Italians let me into their country now. Another year I spent New Year's Eve in Spain. That was wonderful, lots of wine and shrimp and beautiful olive-skinned, black-haired women. Later on that night, we all got in trouble at the officers' club on base. You guessed it! That also involved the military police. They were much nicer in Spain. I only added to the problem when I was late for my plane the next day. The military never could take a joke, especially from an Irishman.

My memories of Christmas and New Year's go back to the 1950s. My father had just died; my mother and I would decorate the tree every year. My brothers would then go out with their dates for the night, leaving my mother and me alone. Every year she and I would stand by the Christmas tree. She would hug me and cry for what seemed an eternity. We would then have a big juicy steak together and go to bed. I wonder how many people have memories like that. I do.

That day was a far cry from my younger days when I found my Christmas presents under the couch. Mother almost killed me. At her wake, a friend said, "You will miss her the most." She was right. Even to this day I miss Mother terribly.

I woke up this morning to snow, not frightful weather, but snow nevertheless. It's beginning to look a lot like you know what. In past years, I'd often been overseas for Christmas. More recently I've been in places like Cortina D'Ampezzo, Innsbrook, Deer Valley, and my precious Sun Valley. People say that all I do is laugh. I do laugh a lot, wouldn't you? I have a lot to be happy about. As we approach Christmas, I expect to be happier. December 21, 2012, is the end of the world in the Mayan calendar. I better hurry up with this book. If something happens, I may be joined by a lot of Irish people in my passing. We'll just have to wait and see. Meanwhile I am busy trying to figure out what to get Nancy for Christmas. I have never had an easy time picking out jewelry. I will figure it out. Irishmen have a way with gifts.

There was one very special Christmas, when my mother took me to see, *The Nativity Story* at Mission Hill Church. It involved another long ride on the trolley. I slept the whole way home, but I still think of that every time I pass the church. It remains special to this day.

Christmas is almost here. I am eagerly waiting for my next doctor's appointment. It could be very important. They may be introducing a new drug that would further slow down the ALS. There are very high hopes for this drug. The doctors don't say much. They don't tell you everything. I guess they don't want to spoil the surprise.

Many times I have been told how ALS can destroy families. It can fracture the family structure. Splits and divorces are common. I now understand how this can happen. ALS just keeps bearing down, causing more damage every step of the way. The pressure, intensity, and uncertainty will wear you down. It has its effect even on a strong relationship like ours. Arguments and disagreements appear where there were none. Now that I can't really talk, misunderstandings are common. This can turn your whole world upside down. It is not easy to be balanced enough to overcome it. Patience, which I was never known for, becomes really important. At this point a very structured and organized life becomes confusing and discouraging.

Now I can almost understand why some people choose not to go on. I'm sure that it can be a very tempting alternative. Not for me. That would be the easy way out. That would be quitting on myself and everyone I ever knew. That won't ever happen. Irishmen don't quit! They must be defeated! In Irish folklore, warriors are respected for their heroism.

I can no longer turn over in bed or pull covers over me. Very recently I have lost my desire to eat. I will have to use the feeding tube now. These changes are among the toughest. At this point, some people elect not to have a feeding tube. As a result they will slowly starve to death. Eventually the increasing levels of morphine kill them. This is basically an assisted suicide, even though it is illegal. No one seems to care. To me it is just plain suicide. At times I have even called it murder. As ugly as it may get, I will go when my breathing stops from natural causes. I told you I was one stubborn Irish bastard!

Nevertheless, Christmas and life go on. Santa will not be denied. There are presents to buy and babies to kiss. Even with awful thoughts running through my head, it is still a joyous time of year. Time to think about Christmas dinner. How does a boneless leg of lamb, red bliss potatoes, cipollini onions, and fennel sound? I'm drooling already. Of course I drool anyway from the disease. Who am I kidding?

I love this time of year. I can't wait to say Merry Christmas to all and to all a good night. I wonder how many Irishmen drool.

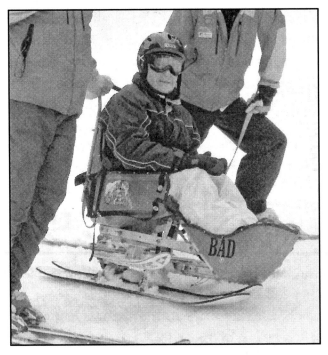

*Richard skiing disabled at the New England Disabled Sport, Loon Mountain.*

Speaking of drooling, I am drooling over the thought of skiing this Saturday, December 15, 2012. Jack Daly has set it up for me at one o'clock. The conditions should be good for this time of year. Everything is getting harder now. The skiing is probably the easiest part. Preparing to leave and the two-and-a-half-hour trip is getting more difficult. The bathroom up north is also more challenging. Overall none of these things are insurmountable.

It is more difficult for Nancy than at home. I hope this does not sound like I am complaining. I'm not. After all it's not like I am camping out. It's a far cry from that. I will persevere. The key is to keep going. I have to remember that I am still normal. The hermit cookies help . Only one week until Christmas now. By the way this Irishman doesn't camp out.


## December 20, 2012


While we were driving to New Hampshire, the news of a tragedy came over the radio. Twenty children and six teachers were massacred by a madman in Connecticut. Man's inhumanity to man can be awful, but this is incomprehensible. This is pure evil, gunning down innocent and good children. I would be lying if I didn't admit I was traumatized by this news. I would rather have given up my life for one of theirs. My angels will constantly pray for them, and their short lives will be remembered forever. I will get back to you after I have a chance to adjust to this tragedy. This weekend will be bittersweet.


## December 23, 2012


I'm back. I am still distraught over Friday's event, but I have a big smile on my face from skiing. I have decided that faith will carry me through everything, no matter how bad. The battle between good and evil will always be with us, but remember, the warriors don't quit. They fight back. I need to put the same blind faith into the rest of my life that I put into skiing. I need to attack the rest of my life like I'm leaning over the tips of my skis and racing down the mountain. In a world filled with both good and evil, that approach is the only one I know.

The New Year is coming; time for new thoughts. I started to daydream about my teenage years and twenties in West Roxbury, a quiet bedroom community west of Boston. Walter Burke came to mind. He was older and a good friend of my brother's. I came to know him as the prince of pranks.

It was the summer between his freshman and sophomore years at Boston College that he got injured. He had a summer job painting with Dickie Donohue. Fooling around on the scaffold, he fell and broke his neck. Because of the work of his doctors, he was not permanently paralyzed. He was left with a stiff neck and a zipper-like incision. While Walter was rehabbing, Dickie's mother visited him to say how sorry she was. In typical Walter fashion, he said, "I'd be fine if your son hadn't pushed me." That is what got Walter started on his way to legend status. Over the years he made a fine art out of not working, which left plenty of time to get into trouble. I'll never forget the time he called my brother's girlfriend's father and told him they were in the car making out at Bellevue Hill. Now that was really stirring the pot. This memory led me to Walter's perennial dream that West Roxbury would get so crazy that the government would invade. Here is how the dream went:

The horizon filled with small, brown puffy shapes. As they approached they became larger and more numerous. Pretty soon the sky darkened as it filled with the brown shapes. Suddenly they were recognizable as brown camouflage parachutes. It was Walter Burke's dream come true. West Roxbury had gotten crazy in a wild ruckus 1960s way. It was out of control, so the government was parachuting psychiatrists in.

This was Walter's crazy dream. He was the perpetual adolescent living his immature frat house life. Life to him was a twenty-four-hour animal-house party. No one ever called Walter a visionary, but he was. He approached life differently. Every social taboo was made to be broken, and he broke them all. A whole generation was about to rebel, and Walter was the point man leading the way. He was a mentor to numerous generations of young athletes, introducing them to wine, women, and song; debauchery at its best. Oh, by the way, he also got many of them college scholarships. Walter had an Irish liver.

Now he lies crying in a bed in a nursing home, left only with his memories of crazy times with Bo Belinsky, Paul Hornung, Dean Chance, and Anita Chu. Now he is on his way out, being given increasing doses of morphine. Sound familiar? The morphine will eventually kill him, opening up a bed for the next victim. Some people call this just enough healthcare. I call it just enough to kill you. Walter deserves better. He is a true Irishman, but a life of wild living has taken its toll on that Irish liver.

## Christmas Eve 2012

Some days I get tired of dying. It is hardest in bed now. I can't roll over or cover myself. I also have trouble breathing. I have no mobility in bed. Once I get up, it is better. I have great mobility with my scooter. On Thursday I will get a more comfortable chair. The VA has saved my butt again.

More than ever I dream about a cure for this awful disease. Eventually, some young researcher will discover the missing protein, making all this seem silly. Something is killing the motor in my motor neurons. At other times I just drift off into the void where my mind seems to escape my paralyzed body. This sounds awful, but it actually feels pretty good. Thank God I still have my mind, as my body marches toward incapacity. I am still not ready to go anywhere yet. I guess some good comes from having an active Irish mind.

As the year ends, it is time to hear Carolyn describe the process:

*Richard sits in his chair and stops every once in a while, looking out into the distance to gather his thoughts, and then he continues. At night he rereads what we've done, and the next day he picks up right where he left off. He is eloquent in his writing . To be a part of Richard's journey has been the experience of a lifetime. There are days that the words he speaks are difficult for him. We usually do the journal later in the day. I can tell it takes more effort to speak the words. I never want to let him down by not understanding him. I try to repeat what he says, and I get upset when I don't get it right away. It's got to be frustrating, and he never makes me feel bad when I don't understand him. God has been good to help me understand him when his voice is just plain tired. Sometimes when we work on the book, I can tell he's exhausted. I always encourage it, though, because I believe it is important for everyone to hear his story.*

## December 26, 2012

Christmas is overshadowed by Walter's death Christmas Eve morning. First my brother; now Walter is gone. The passing of the guard, I guess, although that really happened years ago. Another character is gone. I hope his legend will live on. Not a pretty way to go; too much morphine; no wake; no funeral, just cremation and drop him in a hole. When they say "Life sucks and then you die," they mean it. People sure are crazy. Walter made us all seem a little saner! I hope St. Peter has mercy on him. God knows Walter needs it. His burial plot should be the site of an annual pilgrimage, but I know it won't. People don't care. They are far too busy and self-absorbed.

Walter, I'll see you and my brother on heaven's golf course. It is far nicer than Augusta National. Sadly, another Irishman has been laid to rest.

## New Year's 2012

What did I learn last year from all of this? I learned that those who do not hear, do not listen; those who do not see, do not look. The way to make people happy is to give them what they want, not what you think they should have. Those who are filled with anger and hatred don't deal with it; they spread it. I also learned that there is plenty of love in this world, and I was given lots of it. Time to think about next year, remembering what you plan in January, you realize by December. That's it for this year. I'll be back in 2013.

## January 2013

After skiing in six inches of fresh snow on top of a two-foot base, I am ready to greet this year. My goal is set. I will beat the unbeatable. I will overcome the insurmountable, and I will defeat the inevitable. I will somehow survive! People don't realize that this disease is tailor-made for my attitude. I will treat it like a warrior treats his enemy. I know this is a lot to bite off, but Irishmen have big mouths.

## January 3, 2013

Bad news today. The miracle drug that was so highly touted failed its trial. This news reinforces my feeling that there is no profit in researching and developing a drug for 30,000 people. I wonder how much investment capital they raised by leaking positive information about this drug? Only they know, but the drug failed miserably; that fact should speak for itself. Corporate greed? Who knows? I still hope some young kid will finally find the cure and become a billionaire. As F. Scott Fitzgerald would say, "Living well is the best revenge."

It should be warm this weekend for skiing. I'm looking forward to that. We have also booked a trip to Vail, Colorado, in February. That is another bucket list item. By now you're probably saying to yourself, "What is this guy whining about? Look at all the beautiful places he is going to visit," and you know what? You'd be right. One thing I now realize is that this is not a poor man's disease. Even if you have a lot of resources, it is still tough, but it helps. Lord knows how a person copes who has nothing to fall back on. That is why I am writing this book, to share with others the many phases one's mind has to pass through. It's a journey that never could be imagined. That is also why I spend part of my time raising money and donating to this cause. I don't intend to be the richest man in the graveyard. Contrary to popular belief, Irishmen are not cheap.

I always get wound up before my appointments at Mass General. I feel like I am preparing for a championship boxing match. Physical therapy in the morning. Eat more! Eat more! Eat more! Don't lose any weight! One hundred sixty pounds is where I am now. They don't want me to lose any more. I have to eat more food than I want. Ice cream, too. I have enough Boost to float a ship, and they want me to supplement through my feeding tube. That means more Boost. I hate that word. This is how I became the envy of every woman who has ever had a weight problem. No problem here. It slid off like grease. That's how I am preparing for my next visit to the doctor. Time to make my weight!

No miracle drug to talk about at this next appointment. Wouldn't it be nice if we could talk about improvement in my arms, legs, and voice? This progressive decline is getting old. How do the doctors face this every day? I don't want to sound like Don Quixote tilting at windmills, but I must be optimistic and fight this on my own terms. In the past, when things have gone wrong in life, I always felt as if something would change, and I would find my way out of the mess I was in. I still feel that way. The mess is just a little messier. How's that for stupid Irish optimism?

Breathing is becoming a concern. I also have more mucus forming in my throat. These issues will need to be addressed on Tuesday. One thing about this disease, it is never boring. Something new is always popping up. I really don't know what to expect from this appointment. I can handle almost anything, but I really wish something positive would happen. It's overdue. I guess I'll have to go looking for my lucky Irish shamrock.

## January 15, 2013

I failed to make my weight. This appointment went much as I expected. The downward progression continues, although slowly. My weight is now one hundred fifty-two pounds, a loss of eight pounds. I am going to have to get more serious about the calories. My breathing has also dipped to 38% from 45%. Not good. My ALS assessment score is thirteen, down from twenty-four last year. I wonder what they will do when it is zero and I'm still hanging in there. So much for that assessment tool.

Now for the good news. Overall they seemed to think I am doing great. I have all the equipment I could ever need: computers, lifts, wheelchairs, ramps, and countless other things. The staff members at the MGH and VA have given me great support. For this I am very fortunate and grateful. To tell you the truth, I do get grumpy, but overall I am very happy. It is strange to not be able to use my arms, legs, or voice and still be able to say I feel well. I get tired, but overall I feel great. I am now trying to exercise every day. I hope that will help with the weight problem.

As we write the book, I am now using a communication device part of the time. So far it hasn't slowed us down too much. Like the device, Carolyn even predicts what is coming next.

The truth is that I am really enjoying my retirement, even with this illness. It is over four years now, and I am busier than ever. I can't believe people complain about not having enough to do in retirement. I have enough thoughts in one day to fill a lifetime; so there. I told you Irishmen were dreamers.

After my appointment, we had lunch with the ALS team. They are great, and they always make me feel good. There was a man there who had just been diagnosed with ALS. His wife was crying, and he was terrified. I wanted to talk to him, and I should have. A missed opportunity for sure. The next time I see him, I will make up for it. I will tell him not to give in, and everything will be fine. If I never seen him again, I will not forget that terrified look on his face. He needs a good jolt of Irish optimism.

Last weekend skiing was unbelievable. It was like a dream, spring skiing in January, like skiing on butter. I will ski a few more times before Vail. Planning for a trip is always fun, particularly for Nancy. Boxes are arriving daily at the house. She has already made reservations at Wolfgang Puck's Restaurant, Spago. I will be skiing three days with the adaptive skiing program. New trails are always exciting. The food should be great, even if I can't taste it.

I wish I could take that fellow at the clinic with me to show him what possibilities are still out there for him. The world doesn't stop because of our personal misfortune, thank God. That would be a rough ride. I hope I will have a few good stories when I return. Meanwhile, I will continue my quest to figure out my role in all of this. Not so easy, this business of taking life seriously. It can be hard, but it is worth it. I wouldn't trade my feelings for anything. That's my true heart and soul, a real Irish soul.

I'm waiting for the physicians' report on my last visit. It should be interesting to compare my version with their assessment. Can't wait to see how they characterized it. They do seem to be optimistic though. I now have two machines coming: one for mucus and a nebulizer for improved breathing. These should relieve some of my symptoms. Without a cure, this is all we really do, treat symptoms. These doctors are doing their job. All I have to do is hang in there, so I will trudge through the winter, skiing and eating in style. How's that for confidence? I will let you know what the doctors think. Meanwhile you certainly know how this bloody Irishmen thinks. Such is war.

## January 16, 2013

Billy and I went to the movies today. We saw *Zero Dark 30*, particularly poignant, since his son, Hardy, is a Navy Seal. It was a great movie.

I now realize more than ever that things can always get worse. Just ask Osama Bin Laden. I don't think he is playing golf in heaven. There is a special place for terrorists. Their punishment is to be forever stuck with the seventy seven ugliest virgins ever created. Once that word gets out, there won't be many volunteers. So, God willing, I will live to properly finish this book.

Billy and Sharon are coming over Sunday to watch the Patriots game. I will let you know how it goes. Maybe the Patriots have one more Super Bowl left in them. They don't know how lucky they are to be playing a kid's sport for millions of dollars. The Patriots have come a long way. I remember their very first game in 1960 against the Denver Broncos at Boston University Field.

Barry, Butch, Frank Veino, and I went to the game. We met at the swamp, where Catholic Memorial's football field is now, with two six packs of Heffenreffer Private Stock. We were all fifteen years old. After getting a good buzz, we packed up the rest of the beer and caught the bus from West Roxbury. At Forest Hills we caught the trolley to Brookline Village. It was there that something sacrilegious happened. Butch dropped the beer while getting off the bus. Every last bottle smashed. We all screamed obscenities at Butch as the beer ran into the gutter and down the drain. Barry got so angry he smacked Butch. Butch claims Barry punched him, but he didn't; if he had punched instead of smacked Butch, Butch wouldn't be alive today. To this day I don't think Butch has forgiven Barry. Just so you know, we continued to the game. The Broncos beat the Patriots when Gene Mingo returned a punt for a touchdown. I can still recall every detail of our climbing over the fence at BU field and running past the security guards. They were all about eighty years old. Back then we were mischievous, but not violent. We didn't kill people. If we got angry at someone, we simply sent him a whole slew of magazine subscriptions and made his life miserable.

The Patriots owe us at least one more Super Bowl. Nothing wrong with high expectations. That has allowed me to overcome a lot. I hope it can do the same for them. Look at me; I'm beginning to sound like a blue collar sports fan. Nothing wrong with getting a little jacked up and involved. Maybe it will take Billy's mind off Hardy.

When my brother was dying, I used to make sure the nurses had the Sunday football game on for him. My heart is getting involved now. I'm starting to feel like we're going to crush the Ravens. I better not bet. Go, Pats! I hope there are enough Irishmen on the offensive line. I'll update you on the game Monday, but only if it's good news. Otherwise, I'll be trying to get Billy out of a deep depression.

I recently read about another Christmas death, Billy O'Connor, a fellow St. Theresa's friend and graduate from West Roxbury. In recent years I haven't heard from him. I hope he had a good life. I remember back in church when we sang. Billy and Richard Volke were both blond headed with great voices. My voice sounded like a Mack truck in low gear. I always wondered why God would gyp me like that. The sad thing was that I loved to sing, but I really was bad. Eventually I had to confine my singing to the shower, but Billy will always be remembered, along with my brother and Walter.

The bodies are beginning to pile up. I guess that's part of getting older. We're all like fragile machines that eventually wear out. Maybe that's why I have so many checkups. Have to keep the Irish oil fresh.

## January 21, 2013

This morning a deep depression set over New England. I was wrong. The Pats lost. They really played poorly and didn't deserve to win. As a result I'm going to take a cue from their loss and set my expectations even higher. Guess they never thought of that. I am now determined to make a bigger impact on life and the people around me than ever before. I can now say I am fully committed to living my life in harmony with those around me. It doesn't sound like much, but it takes a lot of awareness and empathy to do it.

This weekend I will ski again in New Hampshire. It has been frigid so far this week, but it should warm up by then. I hope for some more spring-type skiing. Always keep in mind I am not apologizing for my lifestyle. I have earned it, so I will ski as much as I can and leave for Vail on February 10, 2013.

They say death always comes in threes. Sure enough, my cousin Bobby died on January 12, 2013, at the age of eighty-one. Another West Roxbury warrior bites the dust. He was a good man, even though he was half Italian. That part was out of his control. I'll always remember the day he drove me to the hospital when I had pneumonia. I was impressed by his brand new T-Bird at the time. It took two weeks, but I did recover. Another time, he was at one of my football practices when I injured my ankle. Once again he was there to drive me to the hospital. That's the way we were, back then, a close family.

Boy, did his father have a bad temper! God help the cop who dared to pull him over. In another way, a chapter comes to a close with Bobby's death. Thankfully for him he was half Irish.

When I first got the disease, someone told me how much of my life would change because I wouldn't be able to drive. Sure enough, the time came when I could no longer drive. It was different, but it was not the end of the world. We can adapt to most anything. I am now confined to a wheelchair or bed twenty-four hours a day. There is really nothing to fear from this. Life goes on, and we might as well scoot along with it. There is so much adaptive equipment out there that almost anything can be dealt with. If you're new to this disease, have faith and patience, and you will eventually find your way. It's not easy to sort out, but I am living purposefully in what I do every day. I stay true to my plan, even if it's as simple as getting my hair cut. Organization can ease a lot of pain.

I don't consider this a disease really, but an irritation. The most irritating things now are my teeth. The facial muscles have deteriorated to the point they can't fully direct the teeth. As a result, I bite the inside of my mouth, inadvertently causing sores. As weird as it seems, my teeth feel as though they are about to fall out. I hope that doesn't happen before I go to Vail. Now that's a curious symptom, out-of-control teeth. The good news is they are all mine. My message is to anyone who has the disease, legs or no legs, arms and hands or no arms and hands, voice or no voice, there is no reason to give up on what you want to accomplish. It is far too easy to be lazy and blame the disease. The disease can't help itself; we can. In this way, we can all benefit from each other.

Don't be ashamed of anything. Wear your wheelchair like a badge of honor. That chair will allow you to lead a full and happy life, but only if you let it. I'm thinking of painting some Irish shamrocks on mine.

## January 23, 2013

As always, the dogs are looking forward to New Hampshire this weekend. They love the snow! It is time now to give them some credit. Since I have been wheelchair bound, Lexi has been constantly at my side. She is a true service dog and takes her job very seriously. She watches everything I do. She also watches what everyone else does. She can't bear it if I have to leave her home for some reason. She has even started to train Paris, the little monster, to look after me. Paris seems to be getting it. These dogs have a lot of love and empathy. We humans could learn a few things from them.

Time is becoming more of a factor now. As you might have noticed, I am writing more frequently. Not knowing what will come next, I am trying to get in as much as I can before communication gets even harder. All in all, though, we are doing quite well getting everything on paper. The direction of this book is determined by the course of the disease. The road is constantly changing. There will be many more twists and turns. I like to think that I am only halfway through this journey. Time will tell. The pace won't be fast and furious, but it is sure going to be interesting. Meanwhile, hold on and enjoy the ride. Life is constant amazement, and I wouldn't have it any other way.

I now look at the road with wonder and amazement. Beautiful babies and stately maple trees stand out like never before. It is as if

I am seeing idealized images of everything. I was tempted to say a beautiful woman is a beautiful woman, but that has always been the case. I guess lust doesn't count in my idealized world. What a great feeling, though, to see things as they are, without all the filters. It is like being set free. No more imposed perceptions. It is almost like the part in movies where the character enters heaven. Ordinary things take on an aura and brilliance that I haven't seen before. Experiencing this intensity gives me a full appreciation of the world we live in. I think a person needs a lot of time on his hands to experience this. Normally we are far too busy to explore things this deeply. For good or bad, my mind won't shut off, so here I am exploring life. I am determined to find something out, I just don't know what. At times the mystery does seem to open up a bit. I hope I am learning from this journey, and I am not just the victim of a universal bait and switch, which would be too cruel. It would almost be enough to lose hope, but instead I would just let it piss this Irishman off.

It's the dead of winter now, stark and freezing outside. It is time to tell some fireside stories about other characters. The first character is not a person but a place, Charlie's Bar. It was run by big Charlie, little Charlie, and medium Charlie, along with Charlie's wife, Ethel. Charlie's was often the site of Sunday morning egg fights, pitting one generation against another. The characters who were slightly ahead of us in age were always arrogant and remain so to this day. They never did win any egg fights, though.

It was also where most of us made our rite of passage from pimple-faced teenagers to adults, although I admit that not everyone made it through that journey. Bobby Glenn, a Scotsman, once called Charlie's the best bar in the world, and he had been to most of them.

Charlie's wasn't just your average post World War II bar with a bunch of drunks hanging around looking for trouble. It was much more than that.

Everyone always said that West Roxbury was stable because everyone worked for the utilities. That was true, but there was also a mix of doctors, lawyers, politicians, insurance executives, and small-business men; therefore Charlie's had a very intelligent clientele. Literary conversations were more common than sports conversations. These people knew how to give their children the freedom to become individuals, which is why so many success stories have come out of West Roxbury.

I once asked a real old timer why all the old timers drank Old Thompson whiskey. They all had a ball and a bat. To the uninitiated, that is a draft beer and a shot of whiskey. His answer to me was, "We all went away to WPA camps during the Depression. We were building lodges and ski trails for what would become a brand-new industry, recreational skiing. The whiskey up there was bad. When we all got home, the only whisky that tasted that bad was Old Thompson, and it was bad."

Imagine that! They all went away to WPA camps, in order to keep their families together. Guess what? None of them lost their houses, and most of their kids went to college.

Sports were important, but education was more important. That was the key to West Roxbury, and more important, Charlie's. It wasn't just a gathering place. It was also a gathering of like minds to have a few drinks.

It was a unique place. I once brought a college friend there. He marveled at the variety of characters. They were all sitting around drinking and discussing the finer points of Richard Burton's latest movie performance. My friend loved it! The professor was there; he was a school librarian nearing retirement. Uncle Al, the children's pal, was also there. Tall and awkward, he didn't look like much, but he spoke fluent Japanese from the war. I'll never forget how David Sheridan used to piss off little C by calling him "Shortapanta." No matter where in the world anyone went, they always returned to

Charlie's. Nowadays, instead of discussing Richard Burton, they would be watching *Family Feud*. Charlie's was an iconic landmark in West Roxbury. Sadly, it no longer exists. A warriors' gathering place bit the dust, along with all those poignant memories.

## January 28, 2013

It was a cold weekend, but the snow was incredible. I skied Sunday, and everything was very smooth. I even saw John, the bartender from the Common Man, at the mountain. At dinner Sunday night, I again experienced my pet peeve, people who change their table because they don't want to be close to someone who is disabled or sounds different. This seems to happen more often. These people always look and sound the same. The woman is overly coiffed with a sour look on her face. The husband is obsequious to her and not very intelligent. Every time I encounter people of that type, they appear to be nothing but phonies. The good news is nothing can spoil a truly good meal, not even phonies. Oh yes, I almost forgot. Most of the time they also argue over the bill. Judgment time for them will not be pretty. My unsolicited advice to restaurants is to stop serving that type of customer.

Almost time for our Vail trip, only thirteen days away. I consider enjoying life a duty, a true gift that cannot be made up, once it's missed. I drove seniors part-time for a couple of years. The one thing they complained about was being cheated out of their golden years by illness. Truth is, if I can enjoy my golden years, anyone can. No excuses allowed.

I got a new cap to wear in Vail. I still get excited over things like that. My only apprehension about the trip is the length of travel time. I may be putting my Depends to the torture test. The stewardesses are good, but not that good. I will get there, though, and we will have a great time. This Irishman has a lot of willpower.

New England Disabled Skiing at Loon wants me to bring back information on Vail's disabled program. Doing so will make the trip even more interesting. New England has more than two hundred great volunteers. I truly expect Vail's program to be just as professional. The terrain and snow conditions will be a bonus. See, here I go being a kid again. I am easily excited. I am lucky that I have found so many things to do and ways to do them. Modern technology and craftsmanship saves lives like mine every day. I no longer feel like a lone voice in the wilderness crying out for help. Quite the contrary, I am able to be active, independent, and downright ornery. I am making great strides daily in dealing with this disease. Throughout this process I also stayed true to my roots. No phoniness or pretentiousness here, just cold, hard facts. The key to life is living it well, so on I go to Vail. I hope I will get to ski with a lot of Coloradans. Maybe some of them will be Irish. After all, we did help build the cross-country railroad.

One week until we leave for Vail. The Super Bowl was on television, but I pretty much ignored it. Kids are dying in the Middle East and the news is all upset about a blackout at the Super Dome. People are crazy. I hope we aren't abandoning another generation of veterans. We have worn out our military, and it will come back to haunt us. Valor and heroism mean nothing in a superficial world.

My voice is gone now. Even Carolyn has trouble understanding me. I am using the computer to speak more and more. This disability has taught me so much. As a Catholic I now understand the concept of purgatory. Being caught in the constant tension between living and dying is its own purgatory. It is like being in a state of limbo, not knowing what will happen or when.

Thank God I realize that a wheelchair and a bed do not define the boundaries of my world. Even with my limitations I am not going to hold myself back. I am here to fulfill my destiny, with or without all my appendages and faculties. Now I hope you can understand why I am going to Colorado. I am constantly challenging my own will to live. I may not be an Irish warrior physically, but I am one mentally.

## February 5, 2013

My legs are getting very thin and are starting to look deformed. My once-pretty legs are a mere shadow of themselves. I'm lucky that my brother George made me do all those leg exercises when I was a kid. It has probably slowed down the deterioration. Watching the body waste away is probably the hardest part. It takes on the grotesque appearance of someone starving. As the paralysis progresses, my limbs feel like rubber bands that can't be controlled. The mind has a difficult time understanding this. As I head into the more debilitating phase of this illness, I realize that only my mind can rescue me. I know what I have to do. A big part of it is allowing others to help me. I now know the reality of this gruesome disease.

People would think I am crazy if they knew that I truly believe I can outlast this disease. It is a great challenge. Only I can meet it. On day one, I took up a challenge to either beat this affliction or die with dignity trying. Time to tighten up my belly and call myself a wimp if I waver from this path. I have chosen to fight. Already I have put too much into this fight to give up. As long as my mind is willing to battle on, I will never lose my Irish hope or optimism.

## Random Thoughts Before Vail

In case anyone is wondering whether drool pills work, they do. I ran out, and my mouth has been like Niagara Falls. In the morning I wake up and my pillow has a river running through it.

Last night I had a dream about West Roxbury. It centered on Saint Theresa's church. We all went to the eleven o'clock mass and stood in the rear like hooligans. Yes, even Walter would be there. No one ever caught on to the real reason for being in the rear. It was so we could get out early and not wait in line at the donut shop. I had to bring home a dozen, or I was chopped liver.

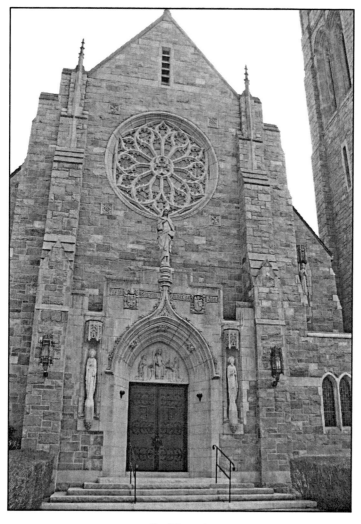

*St. Theresa's*

One Sunday I had my donuts and was passing by Brooks Drugstore on Belgrade Avenue. I noticed fire engines outside Harry Haney's house, another local character. Harry was standing outside on the sidewalk with a big smile on his face. The firemen were carrying Harry's grandfather out of the burning bedroom. Only Lord knows what indignity his grandfather made Harry suffer to deserve this. To this day no one really knows what happened. It's funny how people didn't seem bothered by it.

I don't know why, but I laugh every time I think about it. Characters like him were rampant in those days in West Roxbury. No one ever gave anyone a hard time over anything. The Irish were very, very forgiving back then.

Thoughts about Walter crop up often. He had a paralyzed brother who used a wheelchair. After his parents died, Walter took care of David, and David adored Walter. David knew Walter was crazy, but he still got a kick out of him. That is, until one sunny Saturday afternoon in the fall, when Walter put him out in the back yard to get some sun. Walter then went down to the local tavern for a few beers. Sure enough, everyone was there. Walter drank and bet on the college games all afternoon. Unfortunately he got drunk and forgot all about David. At sundown, someone drove Walter home and found David shivering in the back yard. This memory is not meant to knock Walter. He did a great job taking care of David. Eventually Walter took him to Ft. Lauderdale. Walter called it Ft. Liquordale. David lived out his life in Florida with Walter. Nothing bothered David, because he knew Walter was different. I don't know why I think this story is funny. It must be because I'm in a wheelchair now. There is the constant fear of being in a trapped situation where I can't handle myself. It is like the feeling of helplessness one gets in dreams. I guess I really don't mean that it's funny. Mine is more like nervous laughter. There must be a fine line between cruelty, humor, and fear.

Another story featured Freddy Stanton who was in the army in Pennsylvania. Someone—guess who—called the motor pool and told them to have Freddy drive a car over to meet the general with four tickets to the Army-Navy football game, so off went Freddy, with the culprits, to the game. No one was ever the wiser. So much for Army security!

I almost forgot to tell you about our ninth-grade field trip. I thought Jack Manley planned it all, but he denies it and thinks that I did. I don't know why he wouldn't take credit for the trip.

We rented a bus, and a bunch of us went to the Old Howard Theatre in the West End. After a few beers, we went to see Cupcakes Cassidy do her strip-tease act. Her bra came off, and one breast went stage left and the other went stage right. They were so big that a midget stood on each side to hold them up. It is beyond me why Jack wouldn't take credit for this story.

This will be my final random thought before Vail. It took place in our high school gym. Bob Sawtelle and I were in class practicing high-jump landing and rollovers. We were doing it at about a one-foot elevation. Bob kept fooling around as always. I'll never forget I told him to grow up. His answer was, "Why now? I have the rest of my life." Every so often I think of the fact that he still hasn't made it to adulthood, none of us have. A short time later in gym class, Bob broke his shoulder fooling around. No self-respecting Irish man would ever do that from one foot.

## February 8, 2013: The Blizzard of 2013

Carolyn says that my angels take care of me. Now we are not going to Vail. My doctors put up a stink because of the altitude, 11,000 feet, so we had to cancel our trip, but we will go to New Hampshire after the blizzard. The storm could bring up to three feet of snow in some areas. My flight was canceled anyway, so someone is looking out for me. With the condition of my breathing, there could have been real problems up there. I guess I go overboard on thinking I'm invincible. As a result of this disease I guess I am going to have to be more careful and thoughtful when planning things.

The fact that I have this disease was probably determined at birth. Some would call it my fate, but the way I go through life has not been predetermined. I am free to deal with ALS however I want. Free will and determination belong solely to me. No one realizes how much power that fact gives me over ALS, so my mind tells me forget about Vail and go to New Hampshire with Nancy and celebrate Valentine's Day. Remember, you create your own power from within. I think I'll have an Irish whiskey on Valentine's Day.

## Monday, February 11, 2012

The forecasters were right for a change. The blizzard left over three feet of snow in some places. We were out of heat and power for one night and one morning. The house didn't get too cold, about fifty-five degrees. We had a generator hooked up until we had power.

These are the times one feels useless, confined to a wheelchair. My limitations are greater in an emergency situation. Thoughts of anger, frustration, hatred, dissatisfaction, and pity attack me. I do my best to fight them off, and I think I am winning. My body may be broken, but my spirit is not.

On Wednesday I will drag my broken body to New Hampshire. I will ski, pretending New Hampshire is Colorado and Gypsy Cafe is Wolfgang Puck's Spago. It is nice to have options. Going to Vail at 11,000 feet could have had some serious consequences.

## February 19, 2013

There was tons of snow up North. We had a great Valentine's Day at Gypsy. The Turkish lamb chops were delicious. Great meal, great company.

On Friday I skied. I skied well, even though the snow was getting soft. Halfway through my second run, my guide tripped on thick snow, pulling me down with him. The ski chair rolled over, and I did a perfect face plant. Great move! I only hurt my shoulder, thumb, neck, and leg. Oh, I almost forgot a couple of cuts on my face too. All in all it could have been a lot worse. I think the guide's ego was hurt more than I was. It's good to know I can still take a good crash. It also keeps one humble. This Irishman can crash with the best of them. I didn't shed one tear, either.

Today I received the clinical notes from Mass General.

*Visit Note*
*Patient Name: Flynn, Richard P*

*Date of Visit: January 15, 2013*

*Mr. Flynn returns today in follow-up. He was last seen on October 16, 2012.*

*Since that time he has noted a slight advancement in his symptoms. Swallowing has become more difficult. He is still eating. He does have a feeding tube in place and has occasionally been using it; however, he has not been using it daily. We will likely need to increase use of the feeding tube.*

*He has been bothered by saliva and mucus production. Atropine did not help the saliva, but glycolpyrrolate has effectively managed the saliva. He has tried over-the-counter agents such as Claritin and Benadryl for his mucus. We will recommend saline nebulizers.*

*He has obtained a great deal of equipment through the VA. He has a wheelchair-compatible van as well as electric wheelchair and a DynaVox for communication. He is still skiing through an adaptive program.*

*He uses BiPap at nighttime and if he naps during the daytime.*

*We had a long talk with Mr. Flynn and his wife about a variety of issues. We would like for him to visit today with our speech pathologist regarding nutritional supplementation. He will likely also need Thick-it. We would like for him to visit with our clinic physical therapist. Nursing should also meet with Mr. Flynn. We are going to recommend saline nebulizers. They asked if it was possible to take some of the pills through the feeding tube; this is clearly possible to do.*

*William Samuel David, M.D., Ph.D.*

As you can see, my doctor's assessment was pretty much in line with mine. The mucus and the breathing are the biggest problems now. I am starting to have trouble sleeping, although I'm using all the machines, and they are helping. The final stage of the disease is breathing, so this has me very concerned. I will not be complete if I don't somehow finish this book. My awareness of my progress will always be ahead of my doctor's, because I live it daily.

Now I realize something extraordinary about this disease: the more I embrace it, the more I learn about myself and others. Calm down. This does not mean I am giving up the battle. I will still fight on like an Irish warrior, but I will also go where the disease takes me. I will learn from this experience, and I hope it will help others. My voice is gone now. Only one or two people can understand me. With all the others, I must use the speaking machine. There does seem to be more of a downward progression now, but I'm still determined to accomplish my goals. For some reason I have always felt up to the challenges I face. Even from day one I was very confident. I am still confident that I can survive and learn from this unforgiving illness. It is starting to get uglier, though.

## February 22, 2013

Looking out my dining room window, I can see the barbecue grill. Last week it was completely covered in snow. Normally that would be an indication that spring was coming. A lot of the blizzard snow has melted. The problem is we are expecting another eight to twelve inches this weekend. That's three weekends in a row. Spring won't be here anytime soon.

My breathing continues to get worse. It is more labored now. I have also started to wheeze, and my drooling has increased. It gets worse in bed. I'm not afraid of going to bed at night, but it is more challenging now, as thoughts careen through my head. I can't help thinking that I may not wake up.

The mucus is a real problem now. I can still cough it up, but it is getting harder. I have started getting headaches. They are not bad yet. I've never had headaches before in my life, but I know what is causing them. The weakened breathing at night allows too much carbon dioxide to build up, creating the headaches. I will try to manage the headaches by using the breathing machine during the day, not just at night.

It's unanimous. All my doctors agree that I am stable. Hold on, now, don't get too excited. I think what they mean is that I have been stable more or less between the last two visits. A lack of a lot of new progression is "stable" to them, especially since my breathing has gone from 103 to 38.

The dreams I have now are based on my vulnerabilities. I dream of being on railroad tracks and not being able to get up or in an airplane and the floor falls out from under me or I am in a room alone and the walls are closing in on me. They are all the same general theme. I wake up, and my arms and legs are asleep. Suddenly I realize they are not asleep; they don't work anymore. They are paralyzed, so my dreams have come true. I can't move in bed or talk. To get Nancy's attention, I have to grunt, not so unusual for an Irishman.

I have now lost thirty-three pounds in the last year and a half. The wasting continues. I'm eating more than I have ever eaten in my life. I hope I can stabilize my weight now. That's what I would call stable. All of you overweight women I mentioned earlier, listen up. Stop worrying about your weight. I have lost thirty-three pounds, and no one has told me I look better, so if you are healthy, relax and enjoy your life. Be happy, don't worry, as my Jamaican Irishman would say.

Happy has always been a difficult word for me, like eternity or immortality. What does the word really mean? It means something different for everyone; that's the problem, so I decided to go to the dictionary.

**Happy**

**Definition**

1. **Feeling pleasure**: feeling or showing pleasure, contentment, or joy. "Happy smiling faces"
2. **Causing pleasure**: causing or characterized by pleasure, contentment, or joy. "A happy childhood"
3. **Satisfied**: feeling satisfied that something is right or has been done right. "Are you happy with your performance?"

Not much help. Contented. That sounds like the old milk commercial. Contented cows. *Contented* is not my idea of happy. Back I went to the dictionary.

## Happiness

1. The quality or state of being happy.
2. Good fortune; pleasure; contentment; joy.
   Related forms
   over-happiness, noun

## Synonyms

1, 2. Pleasure, joy, exhilaration, bliss, contentedness, delight, enjoyment, satisfaction.

Happiness, bliss, contentment, and felicity imply an active or passive state of pleasure or pleasurable satisfaction. Happiness results from the possession or attainment of what one considers good: the happiness of visiting one's own family. Bliss is unalloyed happiness or supreme delight: the bliss of perfect companionship. Contentment is a peaceful kind of happiness in which one rests without desires, even though every wish may not have been gratified: contentment in one's surroundings. Felicity is a formal word for happiness of an especially fortunate or intense kind, to wish a young couple felicity in life.

Getting closer, but not really. Most definitions use happy to define happy. How does that work? I guess we are so miserable we can't even define happy or happiness. We are closing in, though:

1. Attainment of what one considers good
2. Bliss is unalloyed happiness.

It's starting to make a little sense, but we are still using the word to define the word. Also, what is good? I could make this same argument for the word *good*, but I won't bore you. None of these descriptions work for me. Happiness is more than delight, satisfaction, or mere pleasure. Happiness to me cuts right to my inner core. Contentment is not good enough. Happiness is having lived my life according to my plan, correctly and meaningfully. How can one be happy without being engaged in something meaningful every day? It leads to a blissful contentment with all you have attempted and attained. It is almost an other-worldly feeling. I don't know how the hell I got here from the word *happy*, but I did. In short, I am very happy with myself and those around me.

The word I have to describe this higher level of happiness is *serenity*. That word captures the essence of my quest to bring meaning and purpose to my life.

I can honestly say I am starting to get it. All the meaning and purpose in life has to come from within. Once you find serenity, everything else follows in its place. This is not a perfect world, but I do understand it a lot better now, confident that my meaning and purpose in life is to use what I have left to the fullest. Accepting this reality leads me to a sense of serenity. Summing this all up, this Irishman can now reveal that he is in a very happy place.

## February 26, 2013

It is not difficult to talk about death now. Like a daily drill, one gets used to it. After six-plus years, I am almost used to the relentless progression of symptoms. This is not to say I like it, but I embrace it for what it is. There is no cure and there is nothing I can do except learn from it. I have learned an awful lot about my body. It is a lot tougher than I realized. I have fallen many times, but I've yet to tear up my knee. My mind has held up better than I imagined. It helps my body through the tough times. I am now in the spontaneous sleep phase. Suddenly I will get very sleepy during the day; this is sort of like narcolepsy, but not as sudden. A nap is needed every day now, along with the breathing machine.

Funny how we miss all the things we take for granted. Every detail now becomes important. Finishing things becomes really important. Loose ends always bothered me, but now it's like a life-and-death struggle to avoid them.

Walking is probably the thing I miss most during the day. You have no idea what I would give to be able to put my hands in my pockets and walk down the street with my old swagger. Wandering aimlessly is what I really miss. The wheelchair is great, but it's not the same.

James Joyce's novel *Ulysses* would have been very different with Leopold Bloom in a wheelchair. Now I have no choice but to complete my Irish odyssey in a wheelchair.

This journal is not meant to be a guide on how to deal with ALS. It is simply a collection of my feelings and thoughts as I react to the reality of the moment. Carolyn, my administrative assistant, gal Friday, and caregiver, has been with me for important stages of this journey. Let's hear how she reacts to these events:

*So now it's been ten months that I've been with Richard. Changes are hard to recognize when you're with someone as much as we are together. It sort of reminds me of when you see your friend's children after only a few weeks and you can't get over how much they've grown, yet they didn't seem to notice.*

*Life is certainly getting more challenging for Richard. His legs have grown weaker in the past few weeks. We were relying on them much more than we realized. Sometimes after a transfer, when his legs give out a little, I always look at him to see his expression. I'm not sure why I do this, but it's become a habit.*

*His ability to speak has changed considerably, but I thank God I still understand about 90% of what he says. When we are working on the book, I catch myself straining to hear his words, and sometimes we have a good laugh at what I think he's said. I need complete silence when we work now. Any little distraction can make it difficult for me.*

*I laugh when I find myself writing the words ahead of their leaving his mouth. I get the biggest kick out of that, when I can predict what he is going to say before he says it. I don't even know if he notices that it happens sometimes.*

*I don't really think much has changed, though. Richard still remains upbeat, and we keep a solid routine every week. People ask me all the time how he is doing, and I always say, "Great." I don't think I am in denial either; he is really doing well. It certainly helps both of us that I can understand him.*

*Richard mentioned that although he can't control any of what is going on with this disease, he has decided to learn from it. I am fascinated how he can stay so positive and make the most of every situation. I, in turn, have learned so much from Richard and his positive attitude. I really believe attitude is everything—not half the battle, everything. We complain about the silliest things. I am the guiltiest. Richard never wakes up in a bad mood, I can't say that. Richard never gets upset if the wheelchair jams in the lift. I can't say I wouldn't. If a beautiful meal arrives and he can't eat it because it's too hard to eat, he doesn't get angry, but I certainly would.*

*It's funny how something like ALS can teach you lessons you would never have learned otherwise. If anyone told me someone could be capable of maintaining a happy life after ALS interrupted it so rudely, I would have serious doubts. It's amazing how powerful the mind can be to accept and overcome this disease. It's not to be believed, some days, the patience Richard has.*

*One day last week, three of us were getting Richard ready for a funeral. All three of us were doing something different to get him ready to leave, and he sat quietly as we did our parts. Part of me watched in awe as he sat patiently. Granted, most days, there is only one person getting him dressed, but there have been some occasions when there were a few of us.*

*Especially in this rush-rush world, we are all running low on patience. It's all about instant gratification. Our coffee wasn't being brewed quickly enough, so someone created the Keurig. We barely mail cards and letters anymore, because it takes too long, so we e-mail. Everything is very fast-paced, which leads me to my next thought.*

*Sometimes it's painful for me to watch my ten-year-old get his cereal in the morning. I am impatient with him. Now I imagine if I had to wait on someone else for literally everything I needed to do, right down to getting out of bed in the morning, and it doesn't stop there.*

*Either Richard is very good at pretending or he has the patience of a saint. He never barks orders; he patiently waits for us to get things ready for him. That attitude has been an eye opener for me. They say God doesn't give you more than you can handle. I really don't know if God said that or not, but I personally don't like that expression. I feel it's a way of justifying that people should handle things that come their way, no matter how tough, and just move on.*

*Richard has actually made me feel differently about that expression these days. His acceptance of the disease and his promise to himself to fight and not give in to pity will be something I'll always have with me. He never goes to "that place" of "what if." He never gets jealous of his friends when they get up and walk out of his house after lunch. He never curses at people in public. He is always kind and considerate. He never speaks poorly of anyone, even those who have acted badly.*

*He takes pleasure in the little things. The dogs really make him laugh, especially Paris, lately. He still loves to go to nice restaurants with Nancy and head up North to go skiing. He loves his get-togethers with friends, old and new. I know he is looking forward to Humarock again soon. I also know he loves writing and can't wait to see this book finished.*

*When Richard speaks of things we take for granted, a whole slew of things came to mind—combing your hair, blowing your nose, pouring a cup of coffee, or just scratching your ear when it's itchy. All these things are now part of the list he speaks of that he no longer can do.*

*Richard has great, loyal friends who love to come over and take him out. They are wonderful guys who would do anything for Richard. They have been a huge blessing. I went to a support meeting for caregivers of ALS patients recently, and some people said those in their lives had disappeared on them after the diagnosis. They stopped calling, stopped visiting, and they had lost all contact. I was shocked.*

*I know everyone deals with things differently, but I was glad that Richard's friends have not deserted him. I do believe people get scared and don't know how to act, but just showing up can make a big difference. Maybe people worry they won't be able to understand the ALS patient, because of the loss of voice, but I wish I could tell them it's okay; they can do the talking.*

*Richard's friends don't always understand him. They make little jokes about it with him. Richard doesn't get angry. He has his computer and iPad to help with communication.*

Carolyn is prejudiced, but her enthusiasm and optimism have helped me push through some very difficult times. Her assistance won't be forgotten. Irishmen have long memories.

Of course speaking is important too, but it can be dealt with through communication devices. The real problem with losing your voice is that you sound weird to yourself. Strange sounds come out of you when you try to speak. Sometimes I can only grunt to get someone's attention. In public this is embarrassing, and people do not react very well. The bad part is that you lose confidence and feel dumb. You lose your self-esteem. One of the biggest obstacles I've had to overcome is my miscommunication with Nancy, something that has been difficult. Warding off these feelings is a daily battle. Miscommunication happens, even though I know my mind has not been affected. If anything, it has improved my intense focus on life and living. Some days I feel like an Irish farmer, struggling to make ends meet and hold the farm together. In a perverse way, everything seems to be making sense. I know that I am headed in the right direction. I am determined to make this work for everyone.

## February 27, 2013

The other day I looked at my hands. They are deformed. The left hand has frozen open. I can't use it at all. My right hand is freezing inward. Exercise has helped slow down the process, so it isn't completely frozen yet. I can still feed myself with my right hand, although it gets messy at times. My right hand is still an important part of my independence.

When I look at these hands, I think of what the sisters at St. Theresa's used to say. "Idle hands are the devil's workshop."

I laugh like hell. What could I have possibly done to deserve this? My hands haven't done anything different from those of the average Joe. I appreciate how important hands are. Even without hands, I'm able to survive. No problem. I'm even going to give it a label, **hands-free living.** For all you pessimists, put that in your Irish pipe and smoke it!

## February 28, 2013

This week we were on the right side of the rain/snow line. No snow, just heavy rain on Sunday and Wednesday. We will be home this weekend for a friend's seventieth birthday, which gives me an excuse to go to the Bridgeway to get a gift certificate for him. I will, of course, have a few Chardonnays.

I'm really pumped up for next weekend. I am racing in the twenty-fourth annual Kostick Kup, a fundraiser for New England Disabled Skiing. Finally some competition. I've missed it so much! Don't ever let anyone tell you that you'll lose your competitive spirit when you get paralyzed. You don't! I'm probably more competitive now than ever. With lots of sleep and a good dose of luck, I may even win an award, and then I would have something to celebrate at dinner. I hope they won't check this Irishman for performance-enhancing drugs.

It is important for me to have you hear Nancy's story. She has been with me from day one. We weren't even married then. She has been totally loyal, and she remains steadfast in her determination to fight this disease alongside me. Here are some of her thoughts:

*Richard has asked me to write something about the changes to him over time, especially the more recent changes, because of his ALS. I am sure as you read Richard's story, you realize what a life-changing experience this diagnosis is for everyone involved, especially if your ALS is considered to be one of the slow-moving ones. Richard has done his best to maintain as normal a life as possible. For the first four years, we were able to do just that. We traveled extensively. Richard had been skiing in Europe for several years before we met. After we met, he had a partner in crime with whom he could share those breathtaking ski areas. I was thrilled to explore the Dolomites with Richard. I had visited Italy several times with my aunt to sight see, but never had been to the mountains. I fell in love with Cortina D'Ampezzo and the surrounding area, but most importantly, I fell in love with Richard. Richard and I also managed to include side trips during each of our ski vacations. Venice became one of our favorite stop-overs. One year we took the train from Venice to Innsbrook, Austria, and even managed to get in a day of skiing while we were there.*

*When traveling to Europe to ski became too daunting, we began to work on Richard's "bucket list." He had started the list when it was confirmed that he did indeed have ALS, so we set our sights on ski resorts in the United States. Richard had dreamed of going to Sun Valley in Idaho since he was a child. He had watched the movie Sun Valley Serenade with Sonja Henie and John Payne. The breathtaking scenery and glamorous characters had stayed in his mind all those years, and he was finally going to experience if for himself (and include me). We loved it so much we returned the following year.*

*Another dream of Richard's that made his bucket list was to ski Deer Valley, Utah, and stay at the famous Stein Erikson Lodge. Definitely another experience of a lifetime; so much to see and so little time to do it in.*

*These days we are content to spend our time skiing in New Hampshire at Loon Mountain. Skiing became more difficult for Richard, but he was not willing to give up his love for skiing, so Richard now skis in what is called the Mountain Man bi-ski (which I call a bucket) and is able to continue to do what he loves most to do—ski. I did ski with Richard his first year of adaptive skiing, but actually felt that I was holding him back. To be honest,*

*I wasn't able to keep up with him, and for my own safety, decided to let him enjoy this pleasure with the wonderful volunteers at Loon's adaptive ski program. Now Alexis and Paris (our two cocker spaniels) and I watch and become mesmerized with the look of joy on Richard's face as he skis down the mountain feeling free of any restrictions that his ALS has put on him.*

*In the last two years, Richard and I have realized what the future holds for us. I don't think we were hiding our heads in the sand, but we didn't want Richard not to live his life to the fullest. His mobility has been declining over the past couple of years. He has gone from walking perfectly and being able to climb stairs without assistance to stumbling a little and walking with a cane to bringing a wheelchair along in case he got tired to being totally wheelchair bound. I do have to say that during this transition, he made sure he was still able to dance with Erika, his daughter, at her wedding. He wouldn't have missed that experience for the world. We also traveled to Ireland, another bucket-list dream, toured the countryside, and even managed to get married on the Cliffs of Moher. God love his friend Bill, who pushed him all the way to the top of the cliff, while Sharon, Father Dara, and I walked it. We never got to see the Cliffs of Moher, because of the mist and the fog, but it sure gave us a memory of a lifetime. Having loved Ireland so much, Richard thought we should join, Sharon and Bill and their family for a return visit and experience the Galway Races. Needless to say, we rented a scooter that trip.*

*Not only has Richard's mobility declined, but his ability to take care of his daily personal needs have become a challenge. He now needs assistance to take a shower and get dressed, take his pills, groom himself, and go to the bathroom. We have hired people to come in during the day to help Richard do all these things.*

*These changes didn't happen overnight. Richard and I have had time to explore all the options available to us, so Richard can continue to live his life to the fullest with courage and dignity. We would never be able to do this alone, knowing very little about ALS. Richard has a strong support system. The Veterans Administration, Compassionate Care ALS, in Falmouth, Massachusetts; The Massachusetts General Hospital ALS Clinic; and his lifelong friends have been there every step of the way. They have educated us, supported us, and provided us with durable goods and medical equipment. But most importantly, they have shown Richard understanding, warmth, and kindness*

*Day-to-day life continually changes for Richard. As time goes on, his ability to swallow, breathe, and eat has become limited. He was advised by his doctors to have a feeding tube placed while it was still safe to do so. He is still able to eat certain foods and drinks 1,100-calorie milkshakes daily, every woman's dream. His doctors are concerned with his continual weight loss and want him to supplement his food using the G tube. We have yet to find a formula that doesn't make him sick to his stomach, though.*

*His breathing is now affected, as his muscles become weaker, causing him to tire very easily. He uses a BiPap at night and a nebulizer several times a day. These do help, but he finds himself needing to take naps during the day to combat fatigue. One of the most debilitating things about the disease is that as the muscles get weaker and weaker, his ability to speak clearly is almost impossible, especially as the day goes on. For Richard it is very frustrating to repeat himself, and most of the time to no avail. His friends, who are very understanding, do their best to decipher what he is trying to say. For those of us who are with him the most, namely Carolyn, who has become like one of our family, and me, it has become increasingly difficult to understand what he is trying to say. Richard still has so much knowledge and wisdom to share with us, and we all realize it is only a matter of time before we will not be able to understand Richard at all. We feel helpless knowing Richard must feel trapped in his own body, and there is nothing we can do to change it.*

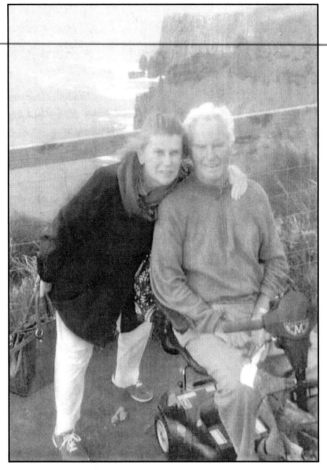

*Richard and Nancy finally get to see the Cliffs of Moher.*

*Richard is now using Assistive Chat, an app that allows Richard to type in what he wants to say, and it will vocalize it for him, but this process will never take the place of hearing Richard's voice and listening to his eloquent way of speaking.*

*Each day brings a new set of challenges to Richard and will continue to do so as his ALS continues to progress. Richard has never been one to give up, no matter the circumstances. He never complains. He continues to be upbeat and positive, and he faces everything head on. There are days he gets discouraged and maybe a "little" grumpy, but given the circumstances, who wouldn't? Despite everything, Richard continues to live his life one day at a time and live it to its fullest. He is an inspiration to everyone he meets. He will never let his ALS get the better of him and beat him down. In Richard's own words, "Irishmen don't ever give up." I just wish I could do more for him other than be there for him daily and love him with all my heart.*

There you have it now, another opinion. We seem to be heading toward a consensus that faith, hope, and determination help in surviving this disease. This Irishman knows one thing for certain: I would cry if I lost Nancy!

## March 1, 2013

Often I think back to the beginning of this journey. To think it all started with one weak finger is hard to believe. If you wanted to defeat an enemy, this is the disease to do it. As I look back, I am most proud of the fact that I never uttered the words, "Why me?" Somehow I knew that was not the answer. To simply start from that point seemed appropriate. At the time it all seemed so random, like balls rolling down a road. Some will veer left, some will veer right, and some will go straight. I think it's called random mathematics. Now it doesn't seem so random. I have been instilled with the strongest sense of purpose and direction in my life. It is hard not to be grateful for this gift. It may seem strange, but that is why I embrace this disease and where it has brought me. I have never been so grounded in my life. My confidence is at an all-time high. Even at this stage I am taking on many new challenges, one of which is this journal. To say that writing this has kept me going would be an understatement. I have been brought to a very good place in life. I am now a master of turning lemons into lemonade. Only a true and faithful Irishman could be this lucky.

<u>**March 2, 2013**</u>

March always reminds me of the national invitational tournament, also known as the NIT. At one time, it was the biggest basketball tournament in the country. College students from around the country converged on New York City for St. Patrick's Day weekend. We were college freshman, and a whole crew of us from West Roxbury went down. It was crazy, drinking and bad behavior everywhere. We stayed at the Commodore Hotel at Grand Central Station, right beside Madison Square Garden. It was wild. Students raised hell all night at the hotel, causing extra security to be alerted.

I'll never forget the next day. We were looking out the window of our seventeenth-floor room when we saw a security guard with binoculars and a two-way walkie-talkie. He was looking for trouble spots. I'm laughing as I remember it. A jackass jumped up and said, "I'll give him a show." He promptly jumped up on the windowsill, hung out the window, and mooned the security guard down below. You should have seen his head swivel as he spotted the culprit and screamed into his walkie-talkie. Moments later, the NYPD burst through the door. They ripped the jackass out of the window, bouncing him off the bed while screaming, "You're probably the son of a bitch that hit me with an ice cube." We were all laughing so hard we were peeing in our pants. The police herded us all into the corridor. Immediately we scattered in all directions down emergency staircases. The NYPD did not pursue us, and neither did we ever return to the room. Like an idiot, I had put the room in my name.

They tried to charge me, and I claimed that some ruffians must have damaged the room after we left.

The year was 1964. Unfortunately we all had far too many weekends like that one. I got home, and all I did was sleep after a five-hour car trip with a guy who had the worst breath ever. I am a bit reluctant to admit it, now that I am sixty-seven years old, but I am that jackass. That Saturday afternoon I almost found out if Irishmen can fly.

Yesterday Billy took me to a lecture on the so-called coffin ships during the Irish potato famine. There were 5,000 of them transporting immigrants to the United States. More than a hundred thousand would die during their voyages. Whole families were given a six-by-six area. With people stacked three high, conditions were deplorable. Waste and human feces were everywhere, and the passengers were not allowed to leave the area. Sometimes the trip took up to sixty days. Being trapped in my own body, I have an understanding of what those passengers must have gone through. Some days I do feel like my body is a coffin as my muscles dry up and wither to nothing. I can only imagine how emaciated and broken those people must have been on arrival in Canada and the United States. How they ever mustered the strength and courage to survive and prosper in their new and sometimes hostile surroundings is beyond me.

They certainly lived, prospered, and produced many offspring. I found out only this week that Butte, Montana, is the most Irish city in the country. Gotcha on that one, didn't I? The reason was the copper mines. Thousands of Irish from Cork emigrated there to work in the mines. It seems the Irish bounce from one disaster to another, a progression not unlike mine. In Butte, they had to deal with lung disease. Many of them died young. To go from one oppression to another seems to be the fate of the Irish. Maybe they shed too many tears in the past to cry now.

## March 4, 2013

I'm looking forward to the race next weekend. I am flying high. I will ski Friday and really go for it Saturday. The race will help soothe thoughts of coffin ships and my frozen coffin-like body. This is one of the biggest races of the year, and I will dedicate my run to those brave Irishmen who died in the belly of a ship searching for a better life.

In my mind this bears similarities to my search for meaning and purpose in my life. During this time I have remained very organized, which has helped me overcome some tough periods. I have been purposeful in all my actions, analyzing every detail and outcome. Racing in the Kostick Kup this weekend is being done for a purpose. I constantly have to challenge my limitations. If not, I will never be able to stand up to this disease. It chews people up. You need to have tough skin to endure it. Any small achievement this weekend will boost my cause.

## March 6, 2013

It takes me a long time to get ready in the morning. As a result I was worried about the early start time at the Kostick Kup. A start time is a lot like a tee time in golf. You can't be late or miss it. You would be disqualified .

Now with another storm bearing down on us, I am more worried about getting up there. We may have to leave on Friday, rather than Thursday.

People ask me if I am afraid of racing. I answer, "No," because I'm not. I was with a friend one night, and I had a disagreement with someone. He threatened to pull a gun on me. I looked him in the eyes and said, "Go ahead, and I'll stick it up your ass." The stranger backed off.

My friend was horrified. He said, "You're crazy."

I answered, "I'm not afraid of him."

My friend's final reaction was, "You're not afraid of anything; that's the problem." I don't think it was meant as a compliment, but I took it as one anyway.

Sometimes my friends ask me what I'm afraid of. My other friend may have been right. I'm not really that sure if I fear anything. I suppose if I had to pick one thing, it would be random violence. I face so much fear every day. Without it, life would not be as challenging. I wouldn't call it an immunity that I have, but fear just doesn't rattle me. I am so used to confronting fear that I have become very resilient. Franklin Roosevelt said, "The only thing we have to fear is fear itself." He was right. We are so busy fearing fear, we can't take action. Me, I just attack it like any other ordinary roadblock in my way.

Over the past seven years, I've become adept at adapting and adjusting to change. Change is ongoing, sort of like those other words, *eternal* and *infinite*. Change must constantly be met and dealt with directly, or it will run right over you. My life now consists of adapting constantly to change and adjusting my activities accordingly. This illness has become the biggest challenge of my life. How I deal with it will determine the meaning of my life. This has become my playing field, and I won't make an error. No one said it was going to be easy, but this Irishman will continue to embrace his fears.

## March 7, 2013

It is Thursday. Sitting here surrounded by snow, sleet, and sideways ice, I realize that I will probably not be going anywhere tomorrow. I hope I'm wrong. It would be two cancellations in eight months. Not a good sign. I hope they will reschedule the race. Time is too short to miss this Kostick Kup.

Yesterday I heard that Rhoda, or actually Valerie Harper, has terminal brain cancer. She has a great attitude. With only three months to live, she is determined to live her life to the fullest. Sound familiar? She is bravely facing her disease head on. This Irishman salutes you, Rhoda/Valerie.

Three months is so little time. No time really to assess her life and realize what is actually going on. This gets back to how lucky I have been to have all this time to organize my thoughts and understand my life more fully. I have been blessed to be able to take a deep and unhurried look at my life. It isn't all pretty, but it's real.

## March 11, 2013

So far this year has been full of disappointments on my end. Last Friday we got hit by another snowstorm, and the driving conditions kept us from going to the Kostick Kup. I was hoping that it would be postponed, but the weather up there was beautiful.

My symptoms are worsening. I have trouble getting enough breaths to blow my nose or clear my throat. My naps are longer and more numerous. In retrospect, it really was a wise decision not to go to Vail. Everything is getting harder, and I am focused on finishing this book by May. What is happening now should not be surprising. It was expected, but I have been spoiled by so many years of doing well. I have to admit this sudden deterioration has blindsided me. How I deal with this will become my legacy. To be truthful, my mind is holding up better that my body. Irish souls must reside in minds, not bodies.

One more trip to go, Turks and Caicos in April, less than a month away now. We have a villa right on the Caribbean. There will be six of us: Nancy, Carolyn, Maggie, Billy, and Sharon, and of course the jackass. Will it be my last trip? Maybe. Maybe not. I'm not telling yet.

You can tell it is trip time, because the packages have started arriving daily. I may look like hell down there, but I will be well dressed. We are setting up restaurants to go to and planning a catered dinner at the villa. Now I don't want to hear any jokes about the last supper. I look at this more like time spent in the desert meditating to my core. I hope I will come back reinvigorated, having adapted once more.

As we head into spring, the reality of this disease bears down on me again. This is not a disease that can be negotiated with by alleviating symptoms. ALS does not play well with others. Like a romance gone bad, it gets under your skin and eats away at you. It is not like an itch you can scratch and be done with it. It marches on, unrelenting in its fury. Like love gone bad, it leaves a sour taste in its wake.

I look back at the beginning now. At first it all seemed harmless and innocent. I really was naïve with regard to where ALS would take me. A journey that began full of hope is turning darker every day. This is not to say I am giving up; it is just reality.

On the darkest days, I look back at my youth. As I look back, brief snapshots of my early life flash before me. Playing ball at Billings Field is always one of them. Hours and hours spent playing ball. Skating through the trees in the swamp is always there too. I was lousy at hockey, but the pickup games were fun. I'll never forget the beautiful young lady from Dorchester who sent me a letter while I was at home, sick in bed. The letter was all about the fine art of French kissing. I read that letter in bed. Later that same summer, she took me into the woods across from her cousins' house and gave me a demonstration. God, was I naïve. At the time that kiss shook me to the core. That was my first taste of city girls.

Every time I hear the song, "You gonna kiss me or not?" I think of that precocious girl from Dorchester. Come to think of it, she may have even been the reason I didn't enter the priesthood.

As I prepare to enter the backstretch of my life, these memories serve me well. They are like a rider's crop spurring me on to the finish line. Whether I win or lose is irrelevant now. To engage in the fight and will myself forward is my priority.

More skiing this weekend. As you might now realize, skiing is more than just a sport or lifestyle to me. Over the years it has become a way to organize my life. It has given me direction and focus when I was veering off course. Skiing has never disappointed me, even when I've gotten lost in Europe and ended up in a new village. Those adventures only add to the mystery of life. Skiing has opened up new vistas for me and allowed me to meet more challenges. Like the motorcycle in *Zen and the Art of Motorcycle Mainten*ance, skiing has given me a clear vision to the world. Unrestrained by framework like a car windshield, the world stretches out before me in its infinite beauty. There's that word again. I am happiest now when I am skiing. That is what happens when you put boundaries and limitations aside. My vision is crystal clear now, and I wake up early every morning excited about the day ahead of me. I never thought I would bond with a disease, but seven years is a long-term relationship, and in many ways skiing has been my savior.

Tomorrow, after my doctor's appointment, I will leave for New Hampshire.

After two hours at the VA, I was too tired to drive to New Hampshire. I am tired a lot now. Feedings, treatments, medication, and machines take up most of my day. One doctor says that I am angry, depressed, and grieving. I say Bullshit! I have never been so busy and active in my life. Honestly I feel really happy. Some days I even reach levels of serenity. Appearance doesn't always match reality.

Getting closer to the end is not easy, but I will deal with my disabilities. I may be deformed, but I am not defeated.

This disease has given me a window of opportunity. I believe I have taken full advantage of it. This has been a long journey, and I have learned much about myself, others, the world, and the universe. One thing I have learned for certain is that some people love you deeply; others love only themselves.

## March 19, 2013

Italians have taught me a lot about love and caring for others. I'll never forget the chairman of the Italian Department at Indiana University. He is a great example. It was 1973, and I needed one more semester of Italian to graduate. It wasn't being offered that final semester. The only option I had was to take a pass-out test. I cringed at the thought.

It was raining cats and dogs as I walked down the corridor to the chairman's office. Not knowing what to expect, I flashed a very weak smile and introduced myself. He was one of the most cordial men I have ever met. After the introduction, he handed me a literary article, sat me down at a desk, and said, "Translate as much as you can in an hour and leave it on my desk."

Believe it or not, it was an article on appearance versus reality by Italian author D'Annunzio. My stomach turned and I almost messed my pants. I said to myself it would be hard in English, never mind Italian. I had no other option, so I reached into my bag of Irish stubbornness and determination and proceeded to plow through the translation, the same qualities I have used against this disease. Very early in the evening two days later, I was there to get my results. As the chairman handed me the results, he invited me to a wine social at his department. I thanked him and said, "I'll see you there." I was afraid to open the envelope. After I arrived home, I finally summoned the courage to open the envelope. What appeared before my eyes was a giant Pass—. What compassion!

That incident began my second love affair; this time it was Italy. Eventually I was able to merge my two loves, skiing and Italy. How lucky was I? As a bonus I can now carry on a conversation in Italian. I think the chairman would be proud.

This weekend we will make one more attempt to ski this year. It will probably be the last weekend for disabled skiing, and then, two weeks from Saturday, we leave for Turks and Caicos. The sun will feel great.

Last night I had trouble sleeping. One story kept coming back to me as I laughed myself to sleep. It involved my brother George, my mother, Freddy Stanton, and of course a seven-year-old me. My sister always left the car keys on top of the radiator in our front hallway. One day it was just too much of a temptation for brother George and Freddy. They gathered me up, and we all went for a joy ride—that is until they saw my mother coming up the street with a bag of groceries in each hand. Her eyes were bulging out, and I swear I could see steam coming out of her head. George and Freddy must have seen the same thing, because they turned the car around so fast they crashed head on into the hydrant in front of the Depetro's house. Adventurers that they were, George and Freddy scattered, leaving behind the key, the steaming car, and me.

My mother was so angry she looked like a crazy Medusa. This very forgiving Irishwoman was very unforgiving that day. Needless to say, George had to wait a long time before he got a car. My punishment was listening to endless stories of how George and Freddy almost killed her baby. Such was life at 42 Chesbrough Road in the 1950s. Very Irish!

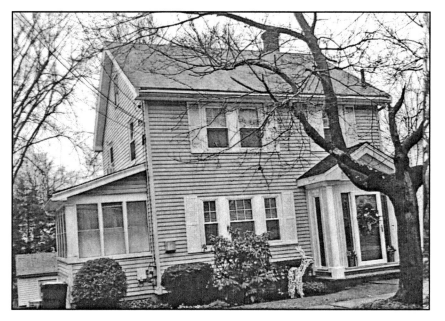

*42 Chesbrough Rd. West Roxbury, MA.*
*Richard was born and spent twenty three years there.*

## March 20, 2013

As I try to prepare for New Hampshire this weekend and Turks and Caicos in two weeks, my daily routine has become stricter. Eating, sleeping, and exercising are the norm.

I expect to die in my sleep, and that is one reason I want to finish this journal by May and publish it in June. The toxin that created this horrendous disease was probably in my body for forty years, maybe as the result of Agent Orange exposure. It simply decided to rear its ugly head in June 2006.

Since then it has been quite the journey. I consider it a journey of recognition and awareness, a re-awakening of my entire universe of thoughts that, like the ALS, lay dormant for years. I hope you have learned as much as I have by taking this journey with me. I now know what I have accomplished and where I am going. I just don't know when. My goal when I started this journal was to give an honest portrayal of my feelings and experiences. Others will decide if I met my own criteria. What surprises me was the enlightenment resulting from this journey of deep exploration. By embracing this disease I have overcome many formidable obstacles and will continue to do so. Originally I was hoping for ten years. It is now seven. Since I am in a good mood today, I am now setting my sights for fifteen. Remember, if you want something, you have to ask. To make this journey has required much faith and hope. It has not been "Two Weeks on the Concord and the Merrimack," but it has been an honest portrayal of my feelings and experiences.


## March 26, 2013


Last Wednesday Loon had eleven inches of fresh snow. On Friday and Saturday it got six more. I skied Saturday in the snow. Great conditions. We had a blast. Cathal, from New England Disabled Skiing in New Hampshire, made my day with this email:

*Nancy,*

*Here is a video of Richard skiing—he is doing a lot of the work himself, and the coach is really only using the tethers for speed control and safety.*

*He is a great example of how to ski that equipment. We enjoyed skiing with him.*

Thank you Cathal! That note only reinforces how I feel about skiing. It makes the time and effort I put in worthwhile. I'm tired all the time now, but skiing invigorates me. I sleep twelve to thirteen hours a night and need a nap during the day. I feel like I am limping to the finish line. I hope I will recover enough energy to carry on.

Skiing's therapeutic value is immense. Without living an active life, skiing and keeping an active mind have allowed me to survive.

## April 2, 2013

Less than a week now to Turks and Caicos. I can picture the villa cascading down a hill to the water. My relationship with Nancy is at an all-time low. We get angry at each other now more than ever. The disease has overwhelmed us. ALS just keeps dragging people down. There won't be much left by the end if we don't find a way to cope with this disease. I think we will all benefit from this vacation.

## Turks and Caicos: April 6 – 13, 2013

As it turns out I was wrong about the villa. It didn't cascade down the hill to the beach. It was right on the beach surrounded by greenery and blooming hibiscus. Everything was on the pool level. It did not disappoint.

The island is a combination of Ernest Hemingway and Graham Greene. Everywhere you look there is hibiscus and bougainvillea.

At the Hemingway Restaurant there were pictures of Hemingway at La Finca, the farm in Cuba. There was also a picture of him on *Pilar*, his favorite boat. Hemingway fished these waters in World War II when he wasn't searching for German U-boats, unauthorized, of course.

The locals were great, and unlike other spots in the Caribbean, the food was great. I had the richest conch chowder ever, with just the right amount of Worcestershire sauce already added. Most unusual. I couldn't eat much food, but I enjoyed watching five other people eat. On Thursday night we had a chef come in and prepare dinner for us. Superb!

The traveling was much more difficult this time. My body has deteriorated to the point that I have to be lifted by people all the time. I am like a 150-pound Raggedy Andy doll. My body has betrayed me. It is a stranger to me now.

On Thursday I did have an adventure. On the way back from lunch, I pulled ahead in my wheelchair and got lost for more than two hours. It was ninety-three degrees out and the sun was blazing hot. As a result I learned two things. Number one, my heart is still strong, and number two, if I didn't get heat stroke that day, I never will. It did improve my tan a lot.

All in all it was a great trip. I feel like a hall-of-fame athlete going out on top, sort of like Ted Williams hitting a home run in his final at bat against Jack Fisher. There is only one problem. With this tan, I no longer look like an Irishman.

It is time now to start shaping the end of this journal. I want to make sure Nancy has a finished product if anything happens to me. If a miracle happens, I will be happy to rewrite the ending. Wouldn't that be something?

Overall I have had a great life, even though I lived through very turbulent times. I have seen many changes in my world. Man landed on the moon. We reached Mars. There were many assassinations. As my brother predicted, the biggest change would be to the phone. I remember back to our front hallway, not far from my sister's keys, there was a mahogany seat and phone table. On it sat a big black rotary phone. The party line came first, and then the two-party line. It was wild. No privacy at all. I can't remember how old I was when we finally got a private line.

Now the communicator in Star Trek has come to life as the cell phone. That and the Internet have changed the way we look at the world. This has been a great era to live through.

I began this journey innocently and probably a bit naïve. The disease has inflicted its damage, and I have the scars to prove it. Thank God I still have my mind, or I never would have gotten this far. This journey is not for the timid. Lou Gehrig said, "I am the luckiest man alive."

This reminds me of just how lucky I am. Lou Gehrig lasted two years. I have already been given seven. Lou had no time to reflect like I have. This has been a great way to get to know myself and others. I hope you have enjoyed my little vignettes from my past. As I progress they bring me a lot of comfort. I have spent much of my life as a loner. I'm not alone now. All of you who read this will make the journey with me.


## March 27, 2013


I think of passing more often now. Society calls it by many names; passing, moving on, and crossing over are among them.

1. **Pass**—intransitive verb, die: to stop living (formal)
2. **Move on**—To leave for elsewhere: to leave a place and go somewhere else, "I think I'll be moving on."
3. **Crossing**—journey across water: a journey across of body of water

In literature, crossing often involves a river. That wouldn't work for me. I'm not a good enough swimmer. Number two works for me. "I think I'll be moving on." That captures the peace and serenity I now feel. When I was a young child, I almost drowned. The memory is vivid. It was a feeling of just slipping away slowly. That time I did pop out of it.

This reminds me of an Emily Dickinson poem. A person was lying in the snow, slowly freezing to death. The poem has almost a pleasurable feeling to it. It seems to capture the same sense of peace and serenity I now feel. That is not to say I enjoy this. I do not, but I have come to terms with my illness. In the end, though, it is all just dying to this Irishman.

My whole body is becoming gaunt and deformed. My arms are really just skin and bones now. My legs aren't much better. My toes are curling under, and my right hand is freezing inward. My voice has very little left.

It has been quite a journey to get to this god-awful point. I still think I can summon the courage to move on for a long time yet. Of course, some days are good and some are bad. Time will tell how far I can go. My future is now!

Some of my doctors think I should cry more; it would help the grieving process. If they only knew I don't cry at all, they would be shocked. God knows I have tried. I lie awake at night and try to cry, but nothing happens. Every so often I think of the afterlife. I don't know what it will bring, but I do know that's my destination. Not being able to cry has kept me strong. One thought to leave you with: Maybe Irishmen don't cry because they can't.

For those of you who have made this journey with me, thank you. You have seen me go from fully capacitated to fully incapacitated. ALS is a soul-crushing disease. I hope you have benefited from this journey. I know I have. ALS has reawakened me. It has restored my fighting Irish spirit and rekindled my interest in my heritage. We have almost come full circle in this long, winding, bumpy, and now rocky road. Not meaning to be morbid, I have tried to talk about death as a natural flow of events. As I look back at the beginning of this journey, so much has changed. My work will continue, and I will continue to write. As far as the rest of my life is concerned, I will continue with the same endless faith and hope I started with. I have met adversity and challenged it. So far I'm happy with my quest for meaning in my life. I couldn't have made that statement seven years ago. It is time now to close out this leg of my journey. After much soul searching, I am in a very good place. It is a loftier place, where even ALS cannot reach me. It is a place where ALS may try to deliver a haymaker, but I am able to deflect it. It is a place where I find serenity. It is a place where anything is possible, including recovery. That place is my mind.

# The End

To end this journal will be difficult. Number one because I'm still alive; number two because everyone already knows the ending. But I will do my best to philosophize a bit about my life. I am long past the time of the predictions given me. That interval has given me a lot of time to think about my own mortality and what the hell my purpose was in being here. I'm not alone in those thoughts, I'm sure.

I think of my mother often. She not only taught me to respect everyone, but she also taught me the principle of reasonableness. All great men are reasonable; otherwise they would not be successful. Reasonableness allows you to dispassionately examine all aspects of a problem. Think of any great leader, and he or she probably had that attribute. I have tried to be reasonable in my daily activities. I haven't always succeeded, but the effort has always been there. Lack of reasoning can create disaster. Robert McNamara, former secretary of Defense, is a great example. History will not be kind to him. He was far too stubborn and intransigent. Time will reveal how many toxic deaths his policies created. Future scholars will expose him for the fraud he was.

Lincoln would be one of my top picks for reasonableness. He would just keep plugging away and changing things until he succeeded. He was also a great businessman. He succeeded on all levels. History may never give this man enough credit. I've always wondered if he had any Irish in him!

Sometimes I let my mind wander and think about my life. I have been blessed and lucky in many ways. I have known many blondes and redheads too, as the song says. I wonder if any of them will be there at the end. I doubt it. I know who will be there, the same people who were always there. After all, we make this journey alone.

I will not take these memories with me. I will leave them all behind. I hope someone will learn something from my experiences. If not, it would be a waste of good effort. Good and bad effort, now that I think about it.

I don't remember much about my father. He was tall with a barrel chest, thin gray hair combed back, and a stern look on his face. He didn't say much. After taking heavy losses early in life, he never really got over them. He was a true accountant through and through. I do remember a Sunday afternoon he took me fishing on the Charles River. It was a sunny day, and we walked over there. We even caught a fish, a big ugly catfish-mackerel-looking thing. Ugly as sin! My father next had a beer or two at what was then called Gagliard's. He was a true Irishmen, right down to the pint of whiskey under his bed.

I also remember the dark Saturday morning he fell in the bathroom with me beside him, never to wake up again. He died that night from a cerebral hemorrhage. I got my sense of detail from my dad. May Saint Patrick bless him!

My brother George and I were the best of friends. I've never before seen a brother-to-brother relationship like ours. Even though we were nine years apart, we were more like twins. We could sense things about each other. He was more like a mentor and second father to me. He introduced me to everything I have done in life, including the beach. Every Sunday afternoon he would take me to the beach, and I would sit between him and his girlfriend. I ruined every Sunday for her. My brother was intelligent, kind, and understanding. I credit him with teaching me how to go after something and get it. At the end I was with him every day. Saint Christopher, guide him through the universe. I miss you, buddy!

I think a lot these days. What do I think about? I think of those around me, and I think of my own mortality. I also obsess with the concept of infinity. It drives me crazy. I realize that only God is immortal. Even as bad as things are, I still don't feel like I am going anywhere soon.

Over the years our goals and aspirations change. When we were children we wanted to be cowboys and Indians, policemen, firemen, and anything else our senses encountered. As we develop, things change. We start to have dreams. I was always a dreamer. At one point I was going to be a priest, but only if I could become pope. How is that for dreaming? I dreamt of faraway places, many of which I have since visited. Traveling became a second love affair behind skiing. My dreams have allowed me to overreach in many ways. I started two companies. I had financial success, went bankrupt, and attained even more financial success after that. One thing I know for certain is that I was never ever afraid to fail. By the way, becoming a priest fell by the wayside when I discovered girls. Being Irish is tough enough.

The universe fascinates me too. It's similar to infinity; it just goes on and on without end. I am awed by the enormity of it all. I even read Stephen Hawking's book, *The Origins of Time*. I was crazy enough to think I understood it. The universe gives me a very spiritual feeling. I am more spiritual now than ever. I feel more closeness with everyone and everything. For a while I thought of getting a spiritual advisor. Writing this book has made it unnecessary. Besides, I have never met a Catholic priest I thought was more spiritual than I am. Catholic priests don't seem to have any interest in helping people. Once the church slipped in this country, it made a decision not to address the problems. It no longer has much of an interest in its parishioners. The church decided to focus all its resources in the southern hemisphere. In essence, the church abandoned its flock, so

I will sit down with my close friends and two bottles of chardonnay and immerse myself in my own homespun spirituality. This spiritual Irishman likes wine, not beer.

The other day I was looking at a picture of Ireland from our first trip. The whole country oozes spirituality. Even our driver blessed himself every time he passed a church. The Catholic Church may have problems in Ireland and the USA, but the Catholic people are just fine.

I looked at one picture, and it was beautiful. It had God written all over it. It reminded me of our wedding; even the ancient pagan Druid ceremony was extremely spiritual. The four basic elements—earth, air, fire, and water—framed the ceremony. Brother Dara loved it!

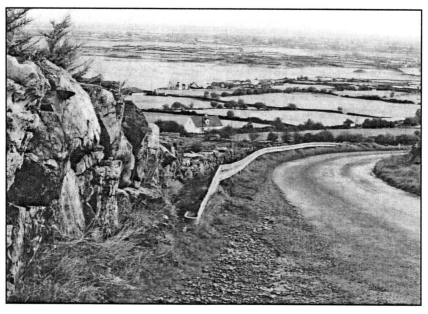

*This picture of Ireland inspired Richard to write this book.*

As I continue this journey, my spiritual side is more pronounced. In many ways, I have been lucky. It is a real blessing to be able to consider your own death for so long a time. People always say they want to die suddenly. I can't think of any worse way to go. I have had plenty of time to consider my own place and purpose for being here. One of the greatest benefits is being able to write this journal. I wonder if a disease has ever been tracked like this before. I hope people can learn from this. Don't give in. Don't ever give in to anything. Get ticked off and get your Irish up, but don't give in!

To die slowly is a real gift. It allows one to reexamine everything over time, including the good and the bad. It is a real rebirth of sorts. I realize very few people ever get the chance to do this. I have. It is almost like being able to relive your life. Winning and losing no longer means as much. The process is more important to me now. I use the principle of reasonableness more than ever. It can be a guiding light when decisions are difficult. It helps create win-win situations. This time has allowed me to assemble my thoughts and delve into why I'm here in the first place. I think I have finally figured it out. Stay tuned. The answer is coming soon. Pay attention, Irishmen!

Man's inhumanity to man has been well documented. I can honestly say that as I get sicker, my fellow man has been very good to me, with few exceptions. Some people have surprised me; others have not. My life has always been an adventure and always will be. I really wouldn't change anything. I've had too much fun the way it is. My only regret is not having a better relationship with my daughter. I have loved her deeply. I remember reading her stories before bedtime. We have both been cheated out of each other. That loss can never me made up. How could it happen? The reality is that it happened. It happens in families every day.

I don't really believe in life being a beginning, middle, and ending, even though because of logic I have written this book that way. Life to me is more of a continuum, passing from one phase to another. I guess, in a way, that's the old dust-to-dust theory. I don't know what my next phase will be, but I do know I am going there with bells on. God help us all if there are no Irishmen there. I know there will be Guinness, so I'm sure there will be an Irishmen or two.

These days I deal with death one day at a time, like an overzealous alcoholic. I don't mean to imply that life has been easy. It hasn't. I've had my share of ups and downs. Life is always hard. It is how you plow through it that counts. Life to me has been wonderful. At my wake I want two songs played: "Silver Thunderbird" by Marc Cohn and "What a Wonderful World" by Louis Armstrong. Louis does a much better job than I do. He sums it all up. Louis should have been Irish.

As my progress continues in this horrible disease, I always come back to this universal question: what the hell am I doing here? I don't think there is any master plan for us. I know, though, that I have fulfilled my destiny. I have lived life to the fullest, without wasting my ability. In fact I think I have overachieved in many areas. In the process I believe I have been good to my fellow man. I have helped others, and others have helped me. I have always tried to do things the right way—some have said to a fault—but at an early age, I learned I do not like doing things the wrong way, no matter what other people do. As I get older and wiser, I realize that this is why I was put here. I have lived my life and used the ability that God gave me.

As far as I'm concerned, I have fulfilled my purpose in life by using my free will to make clear and reasonable decisions. I really don't think I could have done better, and I always refused to cheat. There, I've said it. I have not revealed any secrets to the universe. Sorry. If it seems too simple, it probably is. The key to me has been not to complicate life but to live it. The biggest sin, to me, is not having lived your life to the fullest. Don't waste your time; it is far too precious. I will leave it to those I leave behind to judge what else I have accomplished in life. They will have a much clearer vision than

I. I do think that history will judge me fairly. Saint Patrick wouldn't allow it otherwise.

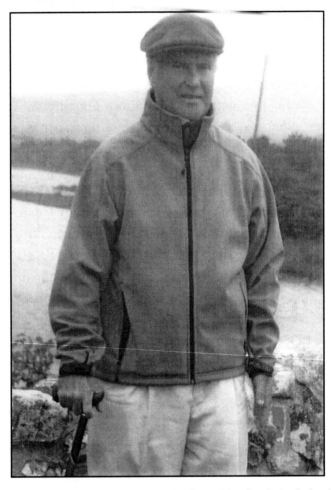

*Richard posing as John Wayne on the Quiet Man Bridge in Ireland.*

This has been an extraordinary journey, complete with a cast of colorful characters. I am no different from anyone else. I was born, lived, and will die. The difference is I've had this time for reflection. Anyone who hasn't should be jealous. It has been quite a gift.

It is now time to talk about Nancy. Whenever anyone would

say something bad about Nancy, her father, Joe, would say, "Not my Nancy." Well, since then, it has become my mantra, "Not my Nancy." She is the last person I see before I go to bed at night and the first person I see every morning. I wouldn't have it any other way.

I don't want to forget the dogs, though. They are there too.

I think it is meaningful to hear what my assistant and caregiver said about Nancy:

*The person who is obviously involved with Richard that I've witnessed consistently is Nancy. She has been selfless in everything. She's constantly watching out for Richard and works very hard to make sure everything is taken care of, making all efforts to see that all his needs are met, appointments are made, and he has all his medicines ready each morning.*

*When I first started working with Richard, sometimes I would overhear him talking to Nancy on the telephone. I used to hear him say, "Whatever you want" at the end of their conversations. I found it sweet, and quite honestly, I was even a bit jealous at times, because phone calls with my husband never quite go like that. But now, after seeing how Nancy puts Richard first, she deserves to hear those words more than anyone.*

*Nancy wakes up and has to face each day with courage, no matter what happens. She never feels sorry for herself, and she never gives up. Nancy is a go-getter and seems to get things done. Richard is very lucky to have her and she him.*

*They complement each other well. She is a great example to all her friends and nieces of what a good wife looks like. I really respect that. Women today don't have the same beliefs about marriage as they did a long time ago, but I love it when I see people who cherish their marriage and each other.*

Every day I grow closer to death. I know it is coming, I just don't know when. I hope you understand from this book that I consider my life a joyous experience. Nancy has elevated it to a higher level. None of this could have been done without her balanced approach to life. I drive her crazy at times, and it just rolls off her. Most of the time she just ignores me until I come to my senses. It will be hard to say good-bye. This book is the only way I know how. I told you a while ago that you all knew the ending ahead of time. You do. I will move on, but this book will live on forever.

Nancy, this book is my love letter to you. *Buona notte, amore mio.* Good night, my love!

CPSIA information can be obtained at www.ICGtesting.com
Printed in the USA
LVOW12s1454220813

348933LV00010B/503/P